D1412937

OXFORD ASSESS AND PROGRESS

Series Editors ·

Kathy Boursicot

Reader in Medical Education and Deputy Head of the Centre for
Medical and Healthcare Education,
St George's, University of London

David Sales

Consultant in Medical Assessment

OXFORD ASSESS AND PROGRESS

CLINICAL
SPECIALTIES

Edited by

Luci Etheridge

Clinical Academic Teaching Fellow in Medical Education,
University College London

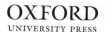

OXFORD
UNIVERSITY PRESS

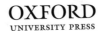

OXFORD

UNIVERSITY PRESS

Great Clarendon Street, Oxford OX2 6DP

Oxford University Press is a department of the University of Oxford.
It furthers the University's objective of excellence in research, scholarship,
and education by publishing worldwide in

Oxford New York

Auckland Cape Town Dar es Salaam Hong Kong Karachi
Kuala Lumpur Madrid Melbourne Mexico City Nairobi
New Delhi Shanghai Taipei Toronto

With offices in

Argentina Austria Brazil Chile Czech Republic France Greece
Guatemala Hungary Italy Japan Poland Portugal Singapore
South Korea Switzerland Thailand Turkey Ukraine Vietnam

Oxford is a registered trade mark of Oxford University Press
in the UK and in certain other countries

Published in the United States
by Oxford University Press Inc., New York

© Oxford University Press 2010

First published 2010
Reprinted 2011, 2012

British Library Cataloguing in Publication Data

Data available

Library of Congress Cataloging-in-Publication Data

Data available

Typeset by Macmillan Publishing Solutions
Printed in China on acid free paper through Asia Pacific Offset

ISBN 978–0–19–956427–9

3 5 7 9 10 8 6 4

SERIES EDITOR PREFACE

The Oxford Assess & Progress Series is a groundbreaking development in the extensive area of self-assessment texts available for medical students. The questions were specifically commissioned for the series, written by practising clinicians, extensively peer reviewed by students and their teachers, and quality assured to ensure that the material is up to date, accurate, and in line with modern testing formats.

The series has a number of unique features and is designed as much as a formative learning resource as a self-assessment one. The questions are constructed to test the same clinical problem-solving skills that we use as practising clinicians, rather than just testing theoretical knowledge, namely:

- Gathering and using data required for clinical judgment
- Choosing examination, investigations, and interpretation of the findings
- Applying knowledge
- Demonstrating diagnostic skills
- Ability to evaluate undifferentiated material
- Ability to prioritize
- Making decisions and demonstrating a structured approach to decision making.

Each question is bedded in reality and is typically presented as a clinical scenario, the content of which have been chosen to reflect the common and important conditions that most doctors are likely to encounter both during their training and in exams! The aim of the series is to build the reader's confidence around recognizing important symptoms and signs and suggesting the most appropriate investigations and management, and in so doing aid development of a clear approach to patient management which can be transferred to the wards.

The content of the series has deliberately been pinned to the relevant Oxford Handbook but in addition has been guided by a blueprint which reflects the themes identified in *Tomorrow's*

Doctors and *Good Medical Practice* to include novel areas such as history taking, recognition of signs including red flags, and professionalism.

Particular attention has been paid to giving learning points and constructive feedback on each question, using clear fact or evidence-based explanations as to why the correct response is right and why the incorrect responses are less appropriate. The question editorials are clearly referenced to the relevant sections of the accompanying Oxford Handbook and/or more widely to medical literature or guidelines. They are designed to guide and motivate the reader, being multi-purpose in nature, covering, for example, exam technique, approaches to difficult subjects, and links between subjects.

Another unique aspect of the series is the element of competency progression from being a relatively inexperienced student to a more experienced junior doctor. We have suggested the following four degrees of difficulty to reflect the level of training so the reader can monitor their own progress over time, namely:

- Graduate should know ★
- Graduate nice to know ★ ★
- Foundation should know ★ ★ ★
- Foundation nice to know. ★ ★ ★ ★

We advise the reader to attempt the questions in blocks as a way of testing knowledge in a clinical context. The series can be treated as a dress rehearsal for life on the ward by using the material to hone clinical acumen and build confidence by encouraging a clear, consistent, and rational approach, proficiency in recognizing and evaluating symptoms and signs, making a rational differential diagnosis, and suggesting appropriate investigations and management.

Adopting such an approach can aid not only being successful in examinations, which really are designed to confirm learning, but more importantly being a good doctor. In this way we can deliver high-quality and safe patient care by recognizing, understanding, and treating common problems, but at the same time remaining alert to the possibility of less likely but potentially catastrophic conditions.

David Sales and Kathy Boursicot, Series Editors
22 May 2009

A NOTE ON SINGLE BEST ANSWER AND EXTENDED MATCHING QUESTIONS

Single best answer questions are currently the format of choice being widely used by most undergraduate and postgraduate knowledge tests, and hence most of the assessment questions in this book follow this format.

Briefly, the single best answer question presents a problem, usually a clinical scenario, before presenting the question itself and a list of five options. Of these five, there is one correct answer and four incorrect options or 'distractors' from which the reader chooses a response.

Extended matching questions are also known as extended matching items and were introduced as a more reliable way of testing knowledge. They are still currently widely used in many undergraduate and postgraduate knowledge tests, and hence are included in this book.

An extended matching question is organized as one list of possible options followed by a set of items, usually clinical scenarios. The correct response to each item must be chosen from the list of options.

All of the questions in this book, which typically are based on an evaluation of symptoms, signs, or results of investigations either as single entities or in combination, are designed to test *reasoning* skills rather than straightforward recall of facts, and use cognitive processes similar to those used in clinical practice.

The peer-reviewed questions are written and edited in accordance with contemporary best assessment practice and their content has been guided by a blueprint pinned to all areas of *Good Medical Practice*, which ensures comprehensive coverage.

The answers and their rationales are evidence based and have been reviewed to ensure that they are absolutely correct.

Incorrect options are selected as being plausible and indeed may look correct to the less knowledgeable reader. When answering questions, readers may wish to use the 'cover' test in which they read the scenario and the question but cover the options.

Kathy Boursicot and David Sales, Series Editors

PREFACE

During the journey through medical school as a student, you experience medicine in a range of settings, from the country general practice to the city teaching hospital. You come across doctors working in a wide range of specialties, many of which will be appealing future career choices and many of which will seem daunting to you. Specialty attachments may be the first time that you encounter people with mental illness, or children, or pregnant women. Trying to absorb all of these new experiences while also continuing to work towards final examinations can seem like a roller coaster ride to some!

In partnership with the well-established *Oxford Handbook of Clinical Specialties*, the *Oxford Assess and Progress Clinical Specialties* volume seeks to tie together the clinical specialties and provide a grounding in knowledge that may get pushed to the back burner when medicine and surgery have to be revised. The questions in each chapter have been written by experienced doctors working within the specialty, familiar with the common presentations, pathologies, and dilemmas that are encountered. Their knowledge of teaching medical students about their specialty, often within the confines of very short attachments, is transferred onto these pages. All questions map onto medical school curricula and are rooted in real-life clinical encounters. The grading system allows you to judge for yourself which knowledge is core and which might require some further reading. The strong focus on clinical experiences also allows you to look forward to your time as a Foundation Doctor.

I hope that, by using these questions, your appreciation and understanding of the different clinical specialties will grow and you will have a useful tool to judge your own learning needs.

Luci Etheridge

ACKNOWLEDGEMENTS

Thanks and gratitude to all contributors, for their hard work at turning their clinical knowledge into questions and providing such thoughtful and considered explanations for readers. For much valued feedback, thanks to all the reviewers, both specialists and students, who have appraised each and every item in the book and provided a unique perspective. Thanks to Dr Jayne Kavanagh for her insightful input on ethical and legal issues. Finally, heartfelt thanks to Caroline Connelly for her inspiration, ideas, and dedication and to Aaron Cue for his continual support.

FIGURE ACKNOWLEDGEMENTS

For Figures 2.1 and 2.6 and all of the figures in the Chapter 7 on dermatology, we are grateful for the permission of Barts and the London NHS Trust for the reproduction of their images and to all patients who consented for images to be used.

Reproduced with permission from Oxford University Press: Plate 2.5: Collier *et al.*, *Oxford Handbook of Clinical Specialties*, 8th edn, p132, Figure 1; Plate 4.1: Sundaram *et al.*, *Training in Opthalmology*, Figure 4.27; Plate 4.2: Sundaram *et al.*, *Training in Opthalmology*, Figure 7.19; Plate 4.3: Sundaram *et al.*, *Training in Opthalmology*, Figure 9.15; Plate 4.4: Sundaram *et al.*, *Training in Opthalmology*, Figure 5.51; Plate 4.5: Sundaram *et al.*, *Training in Opthalmology*, Figure 10.8; Plate 4.6: Sundaram *et al.*, *Training in Opthalmology*, Figure 1.82; Plate 8.1: Hurley *et al.*, *Oxford Handbook for the Foundation Programme*, 2nd edn, p187, Figure 5.

Finally many thanks to all the contributors who supplied images, and to their patients who consented for the images to be used.

CONTENTS

ABOUT THE EDITORS

Volume Editor

Luci Etheridge is a paediatrician by training who currently works as a Clinical Academic Teaching Fellow in Medical Education in the Academic Centre for Medical Education at UCL Medical School. She is involved with the development of Fitness to Practise assessments for the General Medical Council, is an item writer for the Professional and Linguistic Assessments Board Part 1 and the Royal College of Paediatrics and Child Health and runs item writing workshops for UCL Medical School. She is working towards a doctorate in education at the Institute of Education, University of London.

Series Editors

Katharine Boursicot is a Reader in Medical Education and Deputy Head of the Centre for Medical and Healthcare Education at St George's, University of London. Previously she was Head of Assessment at Barts and The London, and Associate Dean for Assessment at Cambridge University School of Clinical Medicine. She is consultant on assessment to several UK medical schools, Royal Medical Colleges and international institutions as well as the General Medical Council PLAB Part 2 Panel and Fitness to Practise clinical skills testing.

David Sales is a general practitioner by training who has been involved in medical assessment for over 20 years, having previously been convenor of the MRCGP knowledge test. He has run item writing workshops for a number of undergraduate medical schools, medical royal colleges and internationally. For the General Medical Council currently he chairs the Professional and Linguistic Assessments Board Part 1 panel and is their consultant on fitness to practise knowledge testing.

CONTRIBUTORS

Dr Erica Allason-Jones NHS consultant in Genitourinary
Medicine, Mortimer Market Centre (Camden PCT), London, UK

Professor Dinesh Bhugra Professor of Mental Health and
Cultural Diversity at the Institute of Psychiatry, King's College,
London, and Honorary Consultant, Maudsley Hospital,
London, UK

Dr Jennifer Birch Consultant in Neonatal Medicine, Luton and
Dunstable NHS Foundation Hospital Trust, Luton, UK

Dr Alex Bonner Specialist Trainee in Anaesthesia and Critical
Care, North West Deanery, UK

Dr Ruth Brown Consultant in Emergency Medicine, St Mary's
Hospital, Imperial College NHS Trust, and Honorary Senior
Lecturer, Imperial College London, UK

Dr Will Coppola Clinical Lecturer and Sub-Dean E-learning,
UCL Medical School, London, UK, and salaried General
Practitioner

Dr Jonathan Darling Senior Lecturer in Paediatrics and
Child Health, University of Leeds, and Honorary Consultant
Paediatrician, Leeds Teaching Hospitals NHS Trust, Leeds, UK

Mr Nev Davies Specialist Registrar in Trauma and
Orthopaedics, Oxford rotation, and Paediatric Orthopaedic
Fellow, Children's Hospital, Westmead, Sydney, Australia

Dr James Dawson Registrar in Anaesthesia and Intensive Care,
Trent Region, UK

Dr Luci Etheridge Clinical Academic Teaching Fellow in
Medical Education, UCL Medical School, and Honorary Specialist
Registrar in Paediatrics, University College London Hospital, UK

Mr Kevin Hayes Senior Lecturer and Consultant in Obstetrics
and Gynaecology, St George's Hospital, London, UK

Dr Kamila Hawthorne GP Principal in Cardiff and Sub Dean for Assessment, School of Medicine, Cardiff University, Cardiff, UK

Dr Virginia Hubbard Consultant Dermatologist, Homerton University Hospital, and Clinical Senior Lecturer, Barts and the London School of Medicine and Dentistry, UK

Dr Vikram Jha Senior Lecturer in Medical Education, Leeds Institute of Medical Education, University of Leeds, and Honorary Consultant Obstetrician, Bradford Teaching Hospitals NHS Trust, UK

Dr Gill MacGauley Reader in Forensic Psychotherapy, St George's University of London, and Consultant in Forensic Psychotherapy, Broadmoor Hospital, West London Mental Health NHS Trust, UK

Dr Matthew Mathai Consultant Paediatrician, Bradford Royal Infirmary, and Honorary Lecturer in Paediatrics and Child Health, University of Leeds, UK

Dr Isobel McMullen Specialty Registrar in Psychiatry, South London and Maudsley NHS Foundation Trust, UK

Dr Zeryab Setna Research Fellow in Medical Education, Leeds Institute of Medical Education, University of Leeds, Leeds, UK

Mr Venki Sundaram Specialty Registrar in Ophthalmology, London Deanery, London, UK

Miss Philippa Tostevin Senior Lecturer in Surgical Education, St George's University of London, and Honorary Consultant Otolaryngologist, St George's Hospital, London, UK

NORMAL AND AVERAGE VALUES

Biochemistry – reference intervals

All laboratory discourse is probabilistic. Drugs may interfere with any chemical method; as these effects may be method dependent, it is difficult for us to be aware of all possibilities. If in doubt, discuss with the lab.

Substance	Specimen	Normal value
Adrenocorticotrophic hormone	P	<80ng/L
Alanine aminotransferase	P	5–35IU/L
Albumin	P†	35–50g/L
Aldosterone	P*	100–500pmol/L
Alkaline phosphatase	P†	30–150IU/L (adults)
α-fetoprotein	S	<10kU/L
α-amylase	P	0–180 Somogyi units/dL
Angiotensin II	P*	5–35pmol/L
Antidiuretic hormone	P	0.9–4.6pmol/L
Aspartate transaminase	P	5–35IU/L
β-HCG	S	M: <10mIU/mL; F (non-pregnant): <25mIU/mL; F (4 weeks pregnant): >1000mIU/mL
Bicarbonate	P†	24–30mmol/L
Bilirubin	P	3–17µmol/L (0.25–1.5mg/100mL
Calcitonin	P	<0.1µg/L
Calcium (ionized)	P	1.0–1.25mmol/L
Calcium (total)	P†	2.12–2.65mmol/L
Chloride	P	95–105mmol/L

(continued)

Cholesterol‡	P	3.9–7.8mmol/L
VLDL	P	0.128–0.645mmol/L
LDL	P	1.55–4.4mmol/L
HDL	P	0.9–1.93mmol/L
Cortisol	P	am: 450–700nmol/L; midnight: 80–280nmol/L
C-reactive protein (CRP)	S	<10mg/L
Creatine kinase	P	M: 25–195IU/L; F:25–170IU/L
Creatinine (related to lean body mass)	P†	70–≤150µmol/L
CSF glucose	CSF	<2/3 of blood range
CSF protein	CSF	<40mg/dL
CSF white cells	CSF	<5/mm³
Ferritin	P	12–200µg/L
Folate	S	2.1µg/L
Follicle-stimulating hormone (FSH)	P/S	2–8U/L (luteal): Ovulatory peak 8–15 U/L Follicular phase, & M: 0.5–5 U/L Post-menopausal: <30 U/L
Gamma-glutamyl transpeptidase	P	M: 11–51IU/L; F: 7–33 IU/L
Glucose (fasting)	P	3.5–5mmol/L
Glycated (glycosylated) haemoglobin	B	5–8%
Growth hormone	P	<20mU/L
Iron	S	M: 14–31µmol/L; F: 11–30µmol/L
Lactate dehydrogenase (LDH)	P	70–250IU/L
Lead	B	<1.8mmol/L
Luteinizing hormone	P/S	Premenopausal: 3–13U/L Follicular: 3–12U/L Ovulatory peak: 20–80U/L Luteal: 3–1 6U/L Post-menopausal: <30U/L

Magnesium	P	0.75–1.05mmol/L
Osmolality	P	278–305mosmol/kg
Parathyrid hormone (PTH)	P	<0.8–8.5pmol/L
Phosphate (inorganic)	P	0.8–1.45mmol/L
Potassium	P	3.5–5.0mmol/L
Prolactin	P	M: <450U/L; F: <600U/L
Prostate-specific antigen	P	0–4ng/mL
Protein (total)	P	60–80g/L
Red cell folate	B	0.36–1.44µmol/L (160–640µg/L)
Renin (erect/recumbent)	P*	2.8–4.5/1.1–2.7pmol/mL/h
Sodium	P†	135–145mmol/L
Thyroid-binding globulin (TBG)	P	7–17mg/L
Thyroid-stimulating hormone (TSH) (normal range widens with age)	P	0.5–5.7mU/L
Thyroxine (T4)	P	70–140nmol/L
Thyroxine (free)	P	9–22pmol/L
Total iron-binding capacity	S	54–75µmol/L
Triglyceride	P	0.55–1.90mmol/L
Tri-iodothyronine	P	1.2–3.0nmol/L
Urea	P†	2.5–6.7mmol/L
Urate	P†	M: 210–480µmol/L; F: 150–390µmol/L
Vitamin B$_{12}$	S	0.13–0.68nmol/L (<150ng/L)

*The sample requires special handling: contact the laboratory.
†Range is significantly different in pregnancy (see below)
‡Desired upper limit of cholesterol would be <5mmol/L.
Key: P = plasma (heparin bottle); S = serum (clotted; no anticoagulant);
B = whole blood (edetic acid (EDTA) bottle); CSF = CSF specimen;
IU = international unit; M = male; F = female;
HDL = high-density lipoprotein; LDL = low-density lipoprotein;
VLDL = very low-density lipoprotein

Arterial blood gasses

pH	7.35–7.45
P_aCO_2	4.7–6.0kPa
P_aO_2	<10.6kPa
Base excess	±2mmol/L

NB: 7.6mmHg = 1kPa (atmospheric pressure≈100kPa)

Haematology – reference intervals

Measurement	Reference interval
White cell count (WCC)	$4.0–11.0 \times 10^9$/L
Red cell count	M: $4.5–6.5 \times 10^{12}$/L; F: $3.9–5.6 \times 10^{12}$/L
Haemoglobin	M: 13.5–18.0g/dL; F: 11.5–16.0g/dL
Packed red cell volume (PCV) or haemocrit	M: 0.4–0.54 I/L; F: 0.37–0.47 I/L
Mean cell volume (MCV)	76–96fL
Mean cell haemoglobin (MCH)	27–32pg
Mean cell haemoglobin concentration (MCHC)	30–36g/dL
Neutrophils	$2.0–7.5 \times 10^9$/L; 40–75% WCC
Lymphocytes	$1.3–3.5 \times 10^9$/L; 20–45%WCC
Eosinophils	$0.04–0.44 \times 10^9$/L; 1–6% WCC
Basophils	$0.0–0.1 \times 10^9$/L; 0–1% WCC
Monocytes	$0.2–0.8 \times 10^9$/L; 2–10% WCC
Platelet count	$150–400 \times 10^9$/L
Reticulocyte count	0.8–2.0% $25–100 \times 10^9$/L
Erythrocyte sedimentation rate	<20mm/h (but depends on age; see OHCM 7th edn p356)
Activated partial thromboplastin time (VIII, IX, XI, XII)	35–45s
Prothrombin time	10–14s

International normalized ratio (INR)	Clinical state (see OHCM, p334–5)
2.0–3.0	Treating deep vein thrombosis (DVT), pulmonary emboli (treat for 3–6 months)
2.5–3.5	Embolism prophylaxis in atrial fibrillation (see OHCM, p335)
3.0–4.5	Recurrent DVT and pulmonary embolism; arterial disease including myocardial infacrtion; arterial grafts; cardiac prosthetic valves (if caged ball, aim for 4–4.9) and grafts

Plasma chemistry in pregnancy

	Non-pregnant		Trimester 1		Trimester 2		Trimester 3	
Centile	2.5	97.5	2.5	97.5	2.5	97.5	2.5	97.5
Na+ (mmol/L)	138	146	135	141	132	140	133	141
Ca^{2+} (mmol/L)	2	2.6	2.3	2.5	2.2	2.2	2.2	2.5
Corrected*	2.3	2.6	2.25	2.57	2.3	2.5	2.3	2.59
Albumin (g/L)	44	50	39	49	36	44	33	41
Free T_4 (pmol/L)	9	23	10	24	9	19	7	17
Free T_3 (pmol/L)	4	9	4	8	4	7	3	5
TSH	0	4	0	1.6	1	1.8	7	7.3

*Calcium corrected for plasma albumin (see OHCM, p670).

Other plasma reference intervals (not analysed by trimester)

	Non-pregnant	Pregnant
Alkaline phosphatase (IU/L)	3–300	Up to 450*
Bicarbonate (mmol/L)	24–30	20–25
Creatinine (umol/L)	70–150	24–68
Urea (mmol/L)	2.5–6.7	2–4.2
Urate (µmol/L)	150–390	100–270

*Occasionally very much higher in apparently normal pregnancies.

- C-reactive protein does not change much in pregnancy.
- TSH may be low in the first half of a normal pregnancy (suppressed by HCG); for other thyroid changes, see above and OHCS 8th edn, p25.
- Protein S falls in pregnancy, so protein S deficiency is difficult to diagnose.
- Activated protein C (APC) resistance is found in 40% of pregnancies so special tests are needed when looking for this. Genotyping for Factor V Leiden and prothrombin G20210A are unaffected by pregnancy.

Paediatric reference intervals

Laboratories vary; consult your own.

	Specimen	Normal value
Biochemistry (1mmol = 1mEq/L)		
Albumin	P	36–48g/dL
Alkaline phosphatase	P	Depends on age*
α1-antitrypsin	P	1.3–3.4g/dL
Ammonium	P	2–25µmol/L; 3–35µg/dL
Amylase	P	70–300U/L
Aspartate aminotransferase	P	<40U/L
Bilirubin	P	2–16µmol/L; 0.1–0.8mg/dL
Bicarbonate	P	21–25mmol/L

Calcium	P	2.25–2.75mmol/L; 9–11mg/dL
Neonates		1.72–2.47mmol/L; 6.9–9.9mg/dL
Chloride	P	98–105mmol/L
Cholesterol	P, F	≤5.7mmol/L; 100–200mg/dL
Creatine kinase	P	<80U/L
Creatinine	P	25–115µmol/L; 0.3–1.3mg/dL
Glucose	F	2.5–5.3mmol/L; 45–95mg/dL (lower in newborn; fluoride tube)
IgA	S	0.8–4.5g/L (low at birth, rising to adult level slowly)
IgG	S	5–18g/L (high at birth, falls, and then rises slowly to adult level)
IgM	S	0.2–2.0g/L (low at birth, rising to adult level by 1 year)
IgE	S	<500U/mL
Iron	S	9–36µmol/L; 50–200µg/dL
Lead	EDTA	<1.75µmol/L; <36µg/dL
Mg^{2+}	P	0.6–1.0mmol/L
Osmolality	P	275–295mosmol/L
Phenylalanine	P	0.04–0.21mmol/L
Potassium (mean)	P	3.5–5.5mmol/L
Protein	P	63–81g/L; 6.3–8.1g/dL
Sodium	P	136–145mmol/L
Transferrin	S	2.5–4.5g/L
Triglycerides	F, S	0.34–1.92mmol/L (30–170mg/dL)

(*continued*)

Urate	P	0.12–0.36mmol/L; 2–6mg/dL
Urea	P	2.5–6.6mmol/L; 15–40mg/dL
Gamma-glutamyl transferase	P	<20U/L
Hormones – a guide (consult laboratory)		
Cortisol	P	9am: 200–700nmol/L Midnight: <140nmol/L (mean)
Dehydroepiandrosterone sulphate	P	Day 5–11 of life: 0.8–2.8µmol/L (range) 5–11yr:0.1–3.6µmol/L
17α-Hydroxyprogesterone	P	Day 5–11 of life: 1.6–7.5nmol/L (range) 4–11yr: 0.4–4.2nmol/L
T_4	P	60–135nmol/L (not neonates)
TSH	P	<5mU/L (higher on days 1–4)

*Alkaline phosphates (U/L): 0–0.5yr 150–600; 0.5–2yr 250–1000; 2–5yr 250–850; 6–7yr 250–1000; 8–9yr 250–750; 10–11yr G = 259–950, B = ≤730; 12–13yr G = 200–750, B = ≤785; 14–15yr G = 170–460, B = 170–970; 16–17yr G = 75–270, B = 125–720: <18yr G = 60–250, B = 50–200.

B = boy, EDTA = edetic acid; F = fasting; G = girl; P = plasma; S = serum.

Haematology (mean ± ~1 standard deviation; range × 10⁹/L (median in parentheses))

	Hb (g/dL)	MCV (fL)	MCHC (%)	Retics (%)	WCC	Neutrophils	Eosins	Lymphs	Monos
Days									
1	19.0 ± 2	119 ± 9	31.6 ± 2	3.2 ± 1	9–30	6–26 (11)	0.02–0.8	2–11	0.4–3.1
4	18.6 ± 2	114 ± 7	32.6 ± 2	1.8 ± 1	9–40				
5	17.6 ± 1	114 ± 9	30.9 ± 2	1.2 ± 0.2					
Weeks									
1–2	17.3 ± 2	112 ± 19	32.1 ± 3	0.5 ± 0.03	5–21	1.5–10 (5)	0.07–0.1	2–17	0.3–2.7
2–3	15.6 ± 3	111 ± 8	33.9 ± 2	0.8 ± 0.6	6–15	1–9.5 (4)	0.07–0.1	2–17	0.2–2.4
4–5	12.7 ± 2	101 ± 8	34.9 ± 2	0.9 ± 0.8	6–15	(4)		(6)	
6–7	12.0 ± 2	105 ± 12	33.8 ± 2	1.2 ± 0.7	6–15	(4)		(6)	
8–9	10.7 ± 1	93 ± 12	34.1 ± 2	1.8 ± 1	6–15	(4)		(6)	
Months (all the following Hb values are medians/ lower limit for normal)									
3	11.5/9	88/88			6–15	(3)		(6)	

(continued)

6	11.5/9	77/70			6–15	(3)		(6)	
12	11.5/9	78/72			6–15	(3)		(6)	
Years									
2	11.5/9	78/74			6–15	(3)		(5)	
4	12.2/10	80/75			6–15	(4)		(4)	
6	13/10.4	82/75			5–15	(4.2)		(3.8)	
12	13.8/11	83/76			4–13	(4.9)		(3.1)	
14B	14.2/12	84/77			4–13	(5)		(3)	
14G	14/11.5								
16B	14.8/12	85/78	30–36	0.8–2	4–13	2–7.5 (5)	0.04–0.4	1.3–3.5	0.2–0.8
16G	14/11.5								
18B	15/13								

Note:
Basophil range: 0–0.1 × 10^9/L; B_{12} (serum): ≥150ng/L.
Red cell folate (EDTA): 100–640ng/mL.
Platelet counts do not vary with age: 150–400 × 10^9/L.
B = boys; G = girls.

ABBREVIATIONS

ABC	Airway, breathing, circulation
ABCDE	Airway, breathing, circulation, disability, exposure
ADHD	Attention deficit hyperactivity disorder
ALS	Advanced Life Support
ASA	American Society of Anesthesiologists
ATLS	Advanced Trauma Life Support
AUDIT	Alcohol Use Disorders Identification Test
BMI	Body mass index
BP	Blood pressure
bpm	Beats per minute
C	Celsius
CD4+	Cluster of differentiation 4
cm	Centimetre
CNS	Central nervous system
CO	Carbon monoxide
CO_2	Carbon dioxide
COPD	Chronic obstructive pulmonary disease
CPAP	Continuous positive airway pressure
CPR	Cardiopulmonary resuscitation
CRP	C-reactive protein
CSF	Cerebrospinal fluid
CT	Computed tomography
CTG	Cardiotocograph
CVP	Central venous pressure
DDH	Developmental dysplasia of the hip
DEXA	Dual energy X-ray absorptiometry
dL	Decilitre
DMSA	Dimercaptosuccinic acid
DVLA	Driver and Vehicle Licensing Agency
ECG	Electrocardiogram
EEG	Electroencephalogram
ENT	Ear, nose, and throat
EOG	*Emergencies in Obstetrics and Gynaecology* (OUP)
ESR	Erythrocyte sedimentation rate

FSH	Follicle-stimulating hormone
FTA-ABS	Fluorescent treponemal antibody absorption test
GABA	Gamma aminobutyric acid
GCS	Glasgow Coma Scale
GGT	Gamma-glutamyl transpeptidase
GI	Gastrointestinal
GMC	General Medical Council
GP	General practitioner
Hb	Haemoglobin
HBcAb	Hepatitis B virus core antibody
HBeAg	Hepatitis B virus e antigen
HBsAb	Hepatitis B virus surface antibody
HBsAg	Hepatitis B virus surface antigen
HBV	Hepatitis B virus
HCG	Human chorionic gonadotropin
Hg	Mercury
HIV	Human immunodeficiency virus
HPV	Human papillomavirus
h	Hour
HRT	Hormone replacement therapy
Hz	Hertz
Ig	Immunoglobulin
IM	Intramuscular
INR	International normalized ratio
IUD	Intrauterine device
IUS	Intrauterine system
IV	Intravenous
IVF	*In vitro* fertilization
kg	Kilogram
L	Litre
LH	Luteinizing hormone
LPA	Lasting Power of Attorney
m	Metre
MAOI	Monoamine oxidase inhibitor
MAST	Military antishock trousers
MCHC	Mean corpuscular haemoglobin concentration
MCNS	Minimal change nephrotic syndrome
MCV	Mean corpuscular volume
MEWS	Modified Early Warning Score
mg	Milligram

μg	Microgram
MI	Myocardial infarction
min	Minute
mL	Millilitre
mm	Millimetre
mmol	Millimole
mph.	Miles per hour
MRI	Magnetic resonance imaging
mU	Milli-units
NICE	National Institute for Health and Clinical Excellence
NSAID	Non-steroidal anti-inflammatory drug
O_2	Oxygen
OHCS	*Oxford Handbook of Clinical Specialties*
ORT	Oral rehydration therapy
PCP	*Pneumocystis carinii* pneumonia
PEP	Post-exposure prophylaxis
P_aO_2	Partial pressure of oxygen in arterial blood
P_aCO_2	Partial pressure of carbon dioxide in arterial blood
PO	Per orum (by mouth)
pCO_2	Partial pressure of carbon dioxide
pO_2	Partial pressure of oxygen
RPR	Rapid plasma reagin
SIGN	Scottish Intercollegiate Guidelines Network
SLE	Systemic lupus erythematosus
SSRI	Selective serotonin reuptake inhibitor
THR	Total hip replacement
TPPA	*Treponema pallidum* particle agglutination
TURP	Transurethral resection of the prostate
U	Unit
UK	United Kingdom
UTI	Urinary tract infection
VDRL	Venereal Disease Research Laboratory
VF	Ventricular fibrillation
VT	Ventricular tachycardia
WHO	World Health Organization
ZIG	Zoster immunoglobulin

HOW TO USE THIS BOOK

Oxford Assess and Progress, Clinical Specialties has been carefully designed to ensure you get the most out of your revision and are prepared for your exams. Here is a brief guide to some of the features and learning tools.

Organization of content

Chapter editorials will help you unpick tricky subjects, and when it's late at night and you need something to remind you why you're doing this, you'll find words of encouragement!

Single Best Answer (SBAs) questions are indicated with this symbol 🔲 and Extended Matching Questions (EMQs) questions with this 🔲. Answers can be found at the end of each chapter. First the SBA answers 🔲, and then the EMQ answers 🔲.

How to read an answer

Unlike other revision guides on the market, this one is crammed full of feedback, so you should understand exactly why each answer is correct, and gain an insight into the common pitfalls.

With every answer there is an explanation of why that particular choice is the most appropriate. For some questions there is additional explanation of why the distracters are less suitable. Where relevant you will also be directed to sources of further information, such as the *Oxford Handbook of Clinical Specialties*, websites and journal articles.

→ http://www.bmj.com/cgi/content/full/334/7583/35?grp = 1

Progression points

The questions in every chapter are ordered by level of difficulty and competence, indicated by the following symbols:

★   *Graduate 'should know'*—you should be aiming to get most of these correct.

★ ★   *Graduate 'nice to know'*—these are a bit tougher but not above your capabilities.

★ ★ ★ *Foundation Doctor 'should know'*—these will
really test your understanding.

★ ★ ★ ★ *Foundation Doctor 'nice to know'*—give these a go
when you're ready to challenge yourself.

Oxford Handbook of Clinical Specialties

The OHCS page references are given with the answers to
some questions. OHCM 8ᵗʰ edn → p340 Please note that this
reference is the 8ᵗʰ Edition of the OHCS, and that subsequent
editions are unlikely to have the same material in exactly the
same place.

The Online Resource Centre

Bonus questions will be released monthly in the run up to final
medical examinations. Visit the website to sign up for alerts as
new questions are added.

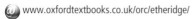 www.oxfordtextbooks.co.uk/orc/etheridge/

CHAPTER 1
OBSTETRICS AND GYNAECOLOGY, AND GENITOURINARY MEDICINE

Erica Allason-Jones, Kevin Hayes, Vikram Jha, and Zeryab Setna

This chapter will be of interest and help to all those studying the healthcare of women. Obstetrics and gynaecology, like all fields of medicine, keeps evolving at a rapid pace, and keeping up to date with the latest literature, guidelines, and protocols can be a daunting task. In the following questions, we have tried to encompass all of the important areas of this subject.

Pregnancy is a joyful experience for both the mother and her family. However, it can occasionally be associated with complications, resulting in severe short- and long-term harm to both the mother and her baby. This chapter covers the most important aspects of pregnancy and its commonly associated problems.

Gynaecological practices are changing constantly, with more emphasis on management in primary care, conservative rather than surgical management of conditions, and an increase in subspecialization, such as gynaecological oncology and urogynaecology. This chapter reflects these changes and covers the most common areas in this interesting field.

Sexual health is a specialty in its own right. The numbers of cases of sexually transmitted infections are rising in the UK, despite efforts to raise awareness of safe sex, so knowledge of their presentations is important. The UK also has the highest rate of teenage pregnancy in Europe, and the Government has set targets to improve access to contraceptive advice for women. In recent years, astounding advances have been made in the treatment of human immunodeficiency virus (HIV) infection and people with HIV can now expect to have a much better quality of life. ∎

Zeryab Setna

OBSTETRICS AND GYNAECOLOGY, AND GENITOURINARY MEDICINE
SINGLE BEST ANSWERS

1. An 18-year-old woman who is 34 weeks pregnant has abdominal pain and moderate fresh vaginal bleeding. The symphysio-fundal height measures 41cm and the uterus feels tense and tender. Her pulse rate is 98bpm and blood pressure is 90/50mmHg. Which is the single most likely diagnosis? ★

A Cervical ectropion

B Placental abruption

C Placenta praevia

D Pre-term labour

E Vasa praevia

2. A 22-year-old woman comes to the antenatal booking clinic at 12 weeks' gestation. Which is the single most appropriate group of booking investigations? ★

A Full blood count, blood group, hepatitis C serology

B Full blood count, blood group, Venereal Disease Research Laboratory (VDRL) test

C Full blood count, thalassaemia screen, thyroid function test

D Full blood count, thalassaemia screen, urea and electrolytes

E Full blood count, thyroid function test, VDRL test

3. A 20-year-old woman and her 23-year-old husband have been trying to conceive for 6 months without success. Her periods are regular. Which is the single most appropriate management? ★

A Arrange a semen analysis for the husband

B Arrange a laparoscopy and dye test for the woman

C Arrange luteal phase progesterone levels for the woman

D Arrange referral to the assisted-conception unit for *in vitro* fertilization (IVF)

E Reassure them and suggest they keep trying

4. A 55-year-old woman has hot flushes. Her last period was 2 years ago. She is keen to start hormone replacement therapy (HRT). Which is the single most appropriate question to ask her before commencing HRT? ★

A Do any of your relatives have Alzheimer's disease?

B Do you know if you have osteoporosis?

C Have any of your relatives suffered from premature menopause?

D Have you ever suffered from deep vein thrombosis?

E Have you ever suffered from depression?

5. A 34-year-old primipara woman is having generalized tonic–clonic convulsions. She is 32 weeks pregnant. Her blood pressure on arrival is 150/110mmHg, she has 3+ proteinuria and she is still having convulsions. The fetal heart is reassuring. Which is the single most appropriate management? ★

A Diazepam and plan delivery

B Diazepam plus antihypertensive and plan delivery

C Magnesium sulphate

D Magnesium sulphate plus antihypertensive

E Magnesium sulphate plus antihypertensive and plan delivery

6. A 23-year-old woman is 34 weeks pregnant and has raised blood pressure. She is on 200mg labetalol twice daily. Her blood pressure is 160/105mmHg and there is 3+ proteinuria. She feels well with no headaches or epigastric pain. The cardiotocograph (CTG) is reassuring. All blood tests are normal. Which is the single most appropriate management? ★

A Admit to hospital for urgent delivery

B Admit to hospital to stabilize blood pressure

C Attend the day unit for twice-daily CTG

D Increase labetalol and follow up with community midwife

E Increase labetalol and follow up in the day unit

7. A 14-year-old girl requests emergency contraception. She had unprotected intercourse 2 days ago with her 14-year-old boyfriend. She appears to understand the nature of emergency contraception. Which is the single most appropriate management? ★

A Advise her that she cannot have emergency contraception as she had intercourse too long ago

B Advise her that she is too young to be legally prescribed emergency contraception

C Prescribe emergency hormonal contraception and advise regarding future contraception

D Prescribe emergency hormonal contraception only after informing her parents

E Prescribe emergency hormonal contraception only after informing social services

8. A 31-year-old woman has vulval soreness and recurrent white vaginal discharge. Microscopy shows the presence of hyphae. Which is the single most appropriate treatment option? ★

A Clindamycin

B Clotrimazole

C Doxycycline

D Erythromycin

E Metronidazole

9. A 35-year-old woman who is taking Cerazette® (a progestogen-only contraceptive pill) has a chest infection and is prescribed amoxicillin. Which single piece of advice should be given about her contraception? ★

A No additional contraceptive precautions are required

B Use additional precautions for the duration of the antibiotic course

C Use additional precautions for the duration of the antibiotic course + 2 days

D Use additional precautions for the duration of the antibiotic course + 7 days

E Use additional precautions for the remainder of the current packet of Cerazette®

10. A 32-year-old primipara is seen at 42 weeks' gestation. She is keen to go into labour naturally and refuses an induction of labour. Which is the single best reason to give for allowing induction of labour when counselling her? ★

A There is increased risk of caesarean section beyond 42 weeks' gestation

B There is increased risk of intrauterine growth restriction beyond 42 weeks' gestation

C There is increased risk of placental abruption beyond 42 weeks' gestation

D There is increased risk of shoulder dystocia beyond 42 weeks' gestation

E There is increased risk of unexplained fetal death beyond 42 weeks' gestation

11. The midwife on delivery suite calls for help. A woman who has just had a normal delivery following active management of the third stage of labour is bleeding heavily. The bleeding started 15min after delivery of the placenta. Her estimated blood loss is 900mL. Her pulse rate is 95bpm and her blood pressure is 100/55mmHg. Which is the single most appropriate first-line management? ★

A Massage the uterus and give IM carboprost (Haemabate®)

B Massage the uterus and give IM syntocinon

C Massage the uterus and start a syntocinon infusion

D Massage the uterus and start a blood transfusion

E Take the woman to theatre immediately for examination under anaesthesia

12. A 32-year-old woman has increasing white vaginal discharge. She is 7 weeks pregnant. Her *Chlamydia* swab is positive. All other tests are normal. Which is the single most appropriate treatment? ★

A Amoxicillin

B Clindamycin

C Doxycycline

D Erythromycin

E Metronidazole

13. A 42-year-old woman has frequency, urgency, and urge incontinence. Examination is unremarkable and a mid-stream specimen of urine is sterile. She is treated empirically for detrusor overactivity with oxybutynin. Which is the single mechanism of action for this drug? ★

A Anti-adrenergic

B AntiGABAergic

C Antimuscarinic

D Antinicotinic

E Antiserotoninergic

14. A 60-year-old woman is recovering post-operatively following a vaginal hysterectomy and anterior vaginal repair. She has had voiding difficulty and has been catheterized for 3 days. A catheter specimen of urine is taken due to a low-grade pyrexia and confirms a urinary tract infection (UTI). Which single organism is most likely to be causative? ★

A *Escherichia coli*

B *Klebsiella pneumoniae*

C *Proteus* species

D *Pseudomonas* species

E *Staphylococcus epidermidis*

15. A 24-year-old woman has had an abnormal vaginal discharge for the past week. It is off-white and non-itchy, with an offensive odour. She has had one sexual partner in the last 8 months and he has no symptoms. There is an off-white vaginal discharge of pH 6.4 pooling in the posterior fornix, with no inflammation of the vulva or vagina. Which is the single most likely finding on a Gram-stained sample of the vaginal discharge? ★

A Gram-negative intracellular diplococci

B Gram-positive and -negative mixed bacteria

C Numerous lactobacilli

D Polymorphonuclear leucocytes

E Yeast cells with hyphae

16. A 24-year-old woman has regular painful uterine contractions at 26 weeks' gestation. She is 2cm dilated. Her membranes are intact. The cardiotocograph (CTG) is reassuring. Which is the single most appropriate management plan? ★

A Admit and administer analgesics and syntocinon

B Admit and administer antibiotics and intramuscular steroids

C Admit and administer antibiotics and tocolytics

D Admit and administer tocolytics and intramuscular steroids

E Reassure and send home

17. A 14-year-old girl has been sexually active for 6 months and seeks sexual health advice. She has a regular partner and has no symptoms. She is very anxious that her mother does not find out that she is sexually active and wants reassurance that her confidentiality will be maintained. In which single situation might breaching her confidentiality be justified? ★

A If she is found to have a sexually transmitted infection

B If she is in a sexually abusive relationship

C If she requests a prescription for the oral contraceptive pill

D If she requests a termination of pregnancy

E None, as she has an absolute right to confidentiality

18. A 25-year-old woman has her first routine cervical cytology test taken as part of the NHS Cervical Screening Programme. This shows 'mild dyskaryosis, CIN 1' and she is advised to have a repeat smear performed in 6 months' time. She has had the same sexual partner for 18 months and they both tested negative for sexually transmitted infections at the start of the relationship. She has a body mass index (BMI) of 30kg/m² and uses a progestogen-only oral contraceptive pill. She smokes 15 cigarettes daily and drinks approximately 25 units of alcohol per week. She wants to know if there is anything she can do that might help the abnormality return to normal. Which single action that she can be advised about is most likely to decrease her risk? ★

A Get vaccinated against human papillomavirus (HPV) infection

B Give up smoking cigarettes

C Reduce alcohol consumption

D Reduce body mass index

E Switch to an alternative contraceptive pill

19. A 24-year-old woman requests post-coital contraception. Her condom broke 36h ago, on day 7 of a regular 29-day cycle. This is her second condom accident in 2 months. She has tried the oral contraceptive pill but stopped it 6 months ago because of concerns about weight gain. She is undecided about future contraceptive use. A pregnancy test is negative. Which is the single most effective form of post-coital contraception for her? ★

A A combined oral oestrogen/progestogen pill

B A progestogen-only pill

C Insertion of a copper-containing intrauterine device (IUD)

D Insertion of a progestogen-containing intrauterine system (IUS)

E No post-coital contraception is required

20. A 27-year-old man has had mild dysuria for 1 week. He has been having sex with his current girlfriend for 4 weeks, occasionally using condoms; she has no symptoms. He last had sex with his previous female partner 3 months ago. There is a slight mucoid discharge at the urethral meatus. Which single organism is the most likely cause? ★

A *Chlamydia trachomatis*

B *Mycoplasma hominis*

C *Neisseria gonorrhoeae*

D *Trichomonas vaginalis*

E *Ureaplasma urealyticum*

21. A 32-year-old man has weight loss and general malaise. He takes an HIV test. The result is positive and his CD4 + count is 180 x 10^6/L (12%) (normal range 450 – 1600 x 10^6/L). He is otherwise well. He does not feel ready to start antiretroviral therapy straight away, but is keen to stay well in the interim. For which single organism should he be offered primary prophylaxis? ★

A *Cryptococcus neoformans*

B *Mycobacterium avium intracellulare*

C *Mycobacterium tuberculosis*

D *Pneumocystis jirovecii*

E *Toxoplasma gondii*

22. A 19-year-old woman has had pain in her vulval area for 4 days. A photograph of the vulval lesion is shown in Plate 1.1. Which is the single most likely diagnosis? ★

A Behçet's disease

B Genital herpes

C Lichen sclerosis

D Syphilitic ulcer

E Vulval cancer

23. A 19-year-old woman has had pain in her vulval area for 4 days. A photograph of the vulval lesion is shown in Plate 1.1. Which is the single most appropriate initial management? ★ ★

A Perform a vulval biopsy

B Prescribe oral aciclovir

C Prescribe oral azithromycin

D Prescribe oral prednisolone

E Prescribe topical clobetasol (Dermovate®)

24. A 26-year-old primigravida is in advanced labour. Her labour has been augmented using syntocinon, so a cardiotocograph (CTG) is performed. This is shown in Plate 1.2. Which is the single most appropriate management? ★ ★

A Perform urgent fetal blood sampling

B Perform an emergency caesarean section

C Reassure the woman

D Stop the CTG recording

E Stop the syntocinon infusion

25. A 29-year-old man from South Africa has collapsed at work. An eye witness gives a clear description of a convulsion. He is drowsy, barely rousable, and unable to communicate. His wife states that she fears he may be HIV positive. His breathing becomes erratic and artificial ventilation is being considered. In which single situation should an HIV test be carried out, given that he is unable to give informed consent? ★ ★

A At the request of his wife, as next of kin

B If knowledge of his HIV status would benefit his care

C Prior to admitting him to the Intensive Therapy Unit

D Prior to any invasive procedure being carried out

E Prior to making the decision to ventilate

26. A 23-year-old woman has a large, 20-week-sized cystic mass on her ovary. She undergoes laparotomy and oophorectomy, and histology confirms that this is a benign mucinous cystadenoma. Which is the single most likely ovarian tissue of origin for this type of cyst? ★ ★

A Epithelial

B Follicular

C Germ cell

D Sex cord

E Stromal

27. A 22-year-old woman who is struggling to conceive has the following hormone profile, taken on day 6 of her cycle:

- Luteinizing hormone (LH): 12IU/mL (normal pre-menopausal 3-13IU/mL)

- Follicle-stimulating hormone (FSH): 4IU/mL (normal 3-20IU/mL)

- Testosterone: 18ng/dL (normal 6-86ng/dL)

An ultrasound scan shows numerous peripheral ovarian follicles. Which single set of symptoms is she most likely to have? ★ ★

A Amenorrhoea and infertility

B Amenorrhoea and pelvic pain

C Oligomenorrhoea and facial hair

D Oligomenorrhoea and pelvic pain

E Oligomenorrhoea and temporal headaches

28. A 24-year-old man who has sex with men has read on the internet that his sexual orientation puts him at risk of hepatitis B virus (HBV) infection. He is interested in being immunized. His hepatitis status results are:

- Hepatitis B virus surface antigen (HBsAg) negative
- Hepatitis B virus core antibody (HBcAb) positive
- Hepatitis B virus surface antibody (HBsAb) negative
- Hepatitis B virus e antigen (HBeAg) negative

Which is the single most appropriate advice regarding his results and proposed immunization? ★ ★

A He has evidence of prior exposure to HBV and is a 'high-risk' carrier; immunization will not help

B He has evidence of prior exposure to HBV and is a 'low-risk carrier'; immunization will not help

C He has evidence of prior exposure to HBV with a partial immune response; immunization is unlikely to help

D He has evidence of prior exposure to HBV with an appropriate immune response; immunization is unnecessary

E He has no evidence of prior exposure to HBV and should proceed with immunization as planned

29. A 16-year-old girl has had painful periods for 6 months. Her periods are regular and last 3 days. She misses a couple of days of school every month due to the pain. She is not sexually active. Which is the single most appropriate initial management? ★

A Combined oral contraceptive pill

B Gonadotrophin-releasing hormone analogues

C Intra-uterine system (Mirena®)

D Mefenamic acid

E Tranexamic acid

30. A 36-year-old woman who is HIV positive discovers that she is pregnant. She is uncertain whether to continue the pregnancy, in particular because of the risk of the child acquiring her HIV infection. Her health is good and she has not yet needed to take antiretroviral therapy. If the pregnancy is managed appropriately, which is the single probability of her baby acquiring HIV infection? ★ ★

A No risk

B Approximately 1%

C Approximately 15%

D Approximately 25%

E Approximately 40%

31. A 26-year-old woman with no children has had amenorrhoea for 6 weeks and has some pelvic discomfort. Her pregnancy test is positive. Her pulse rate is 68bpm and her blood pressure is 110/80mmHg. An ultrasound scan shows an empty uterus, with normal adenexae. Her serum β-human chorionic gonadotrophin (β-HCG) level is 950mIU/mL. Which is the single most appropriate next step in management? ★ ★

A Arrange for a laparoscopy

B Arrange for a laparotomy

C Repeat the β-HCG test in 48h

D Repeat the ultrasound scan and β-HCG test in 48h

E Repeat the ultrasound scan in 48h

32. A 32-year-old primipara woman is 'small for dates' at 34 weeks' gestation. An ultrasound scan shows a singleton fetus with an abdominal circumference at the 10th centile; the amniotic fluid volume and umbilical artery Dopplers are normal. Which is the single most appropriate management? ★ ★

A Cardiotocograph (CTG) monitoring on alternate days

B Reassure her that the baby is growing appropriately

C Repeat the ultrasound scan in 2 weeks' time

D Repeat the ultrasound scan in 4 weeks' time

E Urgent delivery by caesarean section

33. A 30-year-old nurse sustained a significant needle-stick injury during her last shift, 36h ago. The patient ('donor') involved is HIV positive; he is taking antiretroviral therapy and his last viral load was 1000 copies/mL (acceptable <5000 copies/ml). He is hepatitis B virus immune and negative for hepatitis C virus. She also had unprotected sex earlier in her current menstrual cycle and there is a possibility that she may be pregnant. Which is the single most appropriate advice regarding HIV post-exposure prophylaxis (PEP)? ★ ★

A It is already too late for her to start taking PEP

B PEP is contraindicated because of the possibility that she is pregnant

C She does not need PEP as the patient's viral load is so low

D She should start PEP without further delay

E The risks associated with PEP are higher than the risk of acquiring HIV

34. A 37-year-old woman is 15 weeks pregnant and requests a triple test to rule out Down's syndrome. Which is the single most appropriate advice to give her? ★ ★

A It is too early in pregnancy to have the triple test

B It is too late in pregnancy to have the triple test

C She could have the triple test arranged today

D She must first agree to have an amniocentesis if the test is screen positive

E The triple test will definitely be screen positive because of her age

35. A 42-year-old man attends a genitourinary medicine clinic asking for a routine check for sexually transmitted infections. He has no symptoms and no abnormal clinical findings. Serological tests for syphilis show:

- Rapid plasma reagin (RPR) positive at a titre of 1:64

- *Treponema pallidum* particle agglutination (TPPA) assay positive

- Fluorescent treponemal antibody absorption test (FTA-ABS) positive

The same tests were negative 18 months ago. Which single stage of syphilis can be diagnosed? ★ ★

A Early latent

B Late latent

C Primary

D Secondary

E Tertiary

36. A 33-year-old woman has severe headache, blurred vision, abdominal pain, and bleeding per vaginum at 33 weeks' gestation. The fetal heart beat is absent. Which is the single most important associated clinical sign that may help in diagnosis? ★ ★

A Brisk tendon reflexes

B Enlarged thyroid gland

C Oedema

D Raised jugular venous pressure

E Tachycardia

37. A 22-year-old woman is 6–8 weeks pregnant and is brought into the Emergency Department in cardiac arrest. There is no other medical information known about her. Which is the single most likely cause of her cardiac arrest in early pregnancy? ★ ★

A Miscarriage bleeding

B Pre-existing cardiac disease

C Pulmonary embolus

D Ruptured ectopic pregnancy

E Sepsis following termination of pregnancy

38. A 22-year-old woman has acute onset of right iliac fossa pain but no vomiting. She has marked tenderness to palpation in the right iliac fossa. There is no rebound tenderness and some voluntary guarding. Her temperature is 37.2°C, her pulse rate is 80bpm and blood pressure is 115/80mmHg. Her pregnancy test is negative. An ultrasound scan shows a 7cm right-sided haemorrhagic ovarian cyst with no free fluid. Which is the single most appropriate initial management? ★ ★ ★

A Admit with a view to conservative management

B Allow home with advice to come back if pain worsens

C Immediate laparoscopy in case the diagnosis is torsion

D Refer to the surgeons to rule out appendicitis

E Request a computed tomography CT scan to confirm the diagnosis

39. A 70-year-old woman has had vulval itching and discomfort for 12 months. There is widespread erythema on both labia minora extending onto the majora and involving the fourchette. There are no ulcers and no inguinal lymphadenopathy. Which is the single most appropriate initial management? ★ ★ ★

A Empirical treatment with potent corticosteroid ointment

B Immediate punch biopsy to exclude cancer

C Referral to the sexual health clinic to rule out sexually transmitted infection

D Treatment with oestrogen cream for atrophy

E Vulval excision to treat the affected area

40. A 24-year-old woman has dysmenorrhoea and deep dyspareunia. A transvaginal ultrasound scan shows a 4cm endometrioma on the left ovary. She wants improvement in her pain symptoms and also wishes to conceive, as she has been trying for over 12 months. Which is the single most appropriate treatment to use? ★ ★ ★

A Combined oral contraceptive pill

B Danazol

C Gonadotrophin-releasing hormone analogues

D Laparoscopic surgery

E Medroxyprogesterone acetate (Provera®)

41. A previously well 67-year-old woman has abdominal distension, a large irregular pelvic mass and ascites. An ultrasound scan, CT scan, and a raised CA125 confirm a likely ovarian carcinoma. Which is the single most appropriate first-line management? ★ ★ ★

A External beam radiotherapy

B High-dose progestogen therapy

C Hysterectomy, bilateral oophorectomy, omentectomy, and debulking

D Symptomatic palliative care

E Vincristine-containing chemotherapy

42. A 19-year-old woman is on carbamazepine as treatment for her epilepsy. She is 16 weeks pregnant. She had been fit-free for 5 years prior to getting pregnant, but has had two episodes of absence seizures in the past month. She has not informed the Driver and Vehicle Licensing Agency (DVLA) of her recent seizures. Which is the single most appropriate action to take at this stage? ★ ★ ★ ★

A Advise her to inform the DVLA immediately of her recent seizures

B Advise her to seek a second opinion regarding the safety of driving

C Inform the DVLA medical advisor immediately of the recent seizures

D Inform her GP of the recent seizures

E Reassure her that there is no need to inform the DVLA

OBSTETRICS AND GYNAECOLOGY, AND GENITOURINARY MEDICINE
EXTENDED MATCHING QUESTIONS

Causes of testicular problems

For each patient, choose the *single* most appropriate management from the list of options below. Each option may be used once, more than once, or not at all. ★

A Antivirals

B Arrange an ultrasound scan

C Aspiration

D Broad-spectrum antibiotics

E Doxycycline

F Emergency surgical referral

G Penicillin

H Reassurance

I Supportive treatment only

J Urgent urology referral

1. A 19-year-old man has had increasing scrotal pain for the last 24h. He has chills and general malaise. He had painful swellings in his neck and cheeks last week, but these are now improving. He has tenderness of the testis and epididymis on both sides. He has a regular girlfriend, who is well, and always uses condoms during sex.

2. A 17-year-old boy has sudden onset of severe pain in the left side of his scrotum, which came on 2h ago. He says he has had a couple of similar but much milder episodes before, but that these had resolved very quickly. His scrotum is extremely tender on the left. He has had a regular girlfriend for the last 6 months; she is well and they use condoms for contraception.

3. A 26-year-old man has an intermittent swelling in the left side of his scrotum. He first noticed it a year ago and it seems to come and go, being more noticeable when he stands up. It is not painful. When he stands up, there is an ill-defined mobile mass, which feels like a bag of worms, within the scrotum above the left testicle. He has had two sexual partners in the previous 3 months, but used a condom with only one of them.

4. A 24-year-old man has had increasing discomfort in his scrotum for the past 2 days, with some swelling on the right side. The left epididymis is easily palpable and tender, whilst on the right side both epididymis and testis are tender and slightly swollen. There is a small amount of mucoid discharge at the meatus. He started a new sexual relationship 4 weeks ago; his girlfriend is well and is taking the Pill for contraception.

5. A 31-year-old man has a gradual painless swelling of his right testicle. There is a firm lump in the testicle, with no associated tenderness. The lump does not transilluminate. He has been with his current girlfriend for over a year and she is taking the Pill for contraception.

Causes of gynaecological neoplasia

For each clinical scenario, choose the *single* most likely diagnosis from the list of options below. Each option may be used once, more than once, or not at all. ★

A Cervical carcinoma

B Cervical ectropion

C Cervical intraepithelial neoplasia

D Choriocarcinoma

E Endometrial adenocarcinoma

F Endometrial adenoma

G Ovarian cystadenocarcinoma

H Ovarian cystadenoma

I Ovarian dermoid cyst

J Uterine leiomyoma

K Uterine leiomyosarcoma

L Vaginal carcinoma

M Vulval carcinoma

N Vulval intraepithelial neoplasia

O Vulval melanoma

6. A 38-year-old woman has progressive lower-abdominal distension. She has a smooth pelvic-abdominal mass palpable below the umbilicus. An ultrasound scan shows a 10cm simple cystic right-sided mass and no ascites.

7. A 35-year-old para 4 woman has post-coital bleeding. She has a regular 28-day cycle and uses the combined oral contraceptive pill. Her last cervical smear 2 years ago was normal. She has a smooth, centrally red cervix with mild contact bleeding.

8. A 70-year-old woman has had recurrent vulval itching and soreness over the last 12 months that has failed to respond to topical steroid ointments. She has a 2cm ulcerated lesion on the right labium majus.

9. A 30-year-old woman has heavy menstrual bleeding. Her periods are regular and there is no inter-menstrual or post-coital bleeding. She has a bulky 10-week-sized uterus on pelvic examination.

10. A 60-year-old nulliparous woman, whose last menstrual period was 4 years ago, has moderate post-menopausal bleeding. She is obese and has type 2 diabetes. Her last cervical smear, taken 12 months ago, was normal.

Causes of problems in early pregnancy

For each woman, choose the *single* most appropriate next investigation from the list of options below. Each option may be used once, more than once, or not at all. ★

A Amniocentesis

B β-human chorionic gonadotrophin (β-HCG)

C Blood group and rhesus status

D Clotting screen

E Diagnostic laparoscopy

F Full blood count

G Glucose tolerance test

H Serum urea and electrolytes

I Transabdominal ultrasound scan

J Transvaginal ultrasound scan

K Urine for culture and sensitivity

L Urine pregnancy test

11. A 24-year-old primigravida is 10 weeks pregnant. She has frequency of micturition and some dysuria.

12. A 26-year-old primagravida is 10 weeks pregnant. She has marked abdominal tenderness and cervical excitation.

13. A 33-year-old woman is 14 weeks pregnant. She has vaginal bleeding. An ultrasound scan shows a 'snow storm' appearance and no evidence of a fetus.

14. A 23-year-old woman is 7 weeks pregnant. She has been vomiting for the past 2 days. There is a moderate amount of ketones in her urine. Intrauterine pregnancy is confirmed by an ultrasound scan.

15. An 18-year-old woman has had amenorrhea for 8 weeks and now has nausea and generally feels unwell.

Urogynaecological disorders

For each clinical scenario, choose the *single* most likely diagnosis from the list of options below. Each option may be used once, more than once, or not at all. ★

A Bladder stone

B Congenital abnormality of the genitourinary tract

C Cystocele

D Detrusor overactivity

E Enterocele

F Genitourinary tract atrophy

G Genuine stress incontinence

H Interstitial cystitis

I Transitional cell carcinoma of the bladder

J Rectocele

K Urethral stricture

L Urethritis

M Urinary tract infection

N Uterovaginal prolapse

16. A 60-year-old woman has a feeling of 'something coming down' in the vagina. She has no constipation or urinary symptoms. On examination, the cervix is visible on parting the labia.

17. A 60-year-old nulliparous woman has had urinary frequency and urgency for the last 6 months. She occasionally has small 'accidents' before she can get to the toilet.

18. A 16-year-old woman has urinary incontinence almost continuously. It has been going on for years, but she has been too embarrassed to talk about it before. She has a moist vulva and vagina and there is a central thin vaginal septum. There is no stress incontinence on coughing.

19. A 28-year-old woman has urinary frequency and dysuria. An endocervical swab is positive for *Chlamydia trachomatis*.

20. A 63-year-old woman has had urinary frequency, dysuria, and dyspareunia for the last 6 months. Her symptoms markedly improve with local estradiol cream.

Causes of problems in pregnancy

For each patient, choose the *single* most likely diagnosis from the list of options below. Each option may be used once, more than once, or not at all. ★

A Asthma

B Deep vein thrombosis

C Eclampsia

D Epilepsy

E Essential hypertension

F Gestational diabetes

G Hypothyroidism

H Iron-deficiency anaemia

I Migraine

J Myocardial infarction

K Pancreatitis

L Pre-eclampsia

M Pulmonary embolism

N Thalassaemia

O Urinary tract infection

21. A 30-year-old unbooked primigravida has delivered a 4.7kg baby at 36 weeks' gestation. There was difficulty in delivering the shoulders (shoulder dystocia).

22. An 18-year-old primagravida at 36 weeks' gestation has severe epigastric pain and headache. Her pulse rate is 80bpm and her blood pressure is 140/98mmHg. A urine dipstick test shows 2+ proteinuria.

23. A 36-year-old para 4 woman is 35 weeks pregnant. She has sudden onset of shortness of breath. Her pulse rate is 100bpm, blood pressure is 100/70mmHg, and her oxygen saturation is 94% on air. She has recently had a sprained ankle, as a result of which she has had restricted mobility.

24. A 31-year-old para 6 woman books in to the antenatal clinic. Her last delivery was 6 months ago. She feels tired and weak. She has a haemoglobin (Hb) level of 7.3g/dL, a mean corpuscular volume (MCV) of 69 fL, and a mean cell Hb concentration (MCHC) of 30g/dL.

25. A 25-year-old primigravida at 36 weeks' gestation has two episodes of tonic–clonic seizures and is confused. Her pulse rate is 78bpm, blood pressure is 110/70mmHg, and oxygen saturation is 98% on air. A urine dipstick test shows 3+ proteinuria.

Single Best Answers

1. B ★ OHCS 8th edn → p56

This woman is shocked. The abdominal pain and tense uterus suggest abruption. Blood loss may be concealed so do not expect large amounts of visible bleeding. Placenta praevia is usually painless and the blood loss larger so is often noticed earlier. There are no contractions so labour has not started, although delivery will be expedited as she is unwell. A cervical ectropion may bleed but will not cause pain and shock.

2. B ★ OHCS 8th edn → p8

→ http://www.nice.org.uk/nicemedia/pdf/CG062NICEguideline.pdf

3. E ★ OHCS 8th edn → p292

Normal healthy couples can take a year to conceive so investigations are not normally started until after 1 year of regularly trying.

4. D ★ OHCS 8th edn → p257

Overall, HRT doubles the risk of venous thromboembolism so other risk factors need to be considered. HRT helps reduce the risk of fractures in osteoporosis. There is no association with Alzheimer's disease; in fact, HRT may be protective. In some women, symptoms of depression may occur with some forms of HRT, but this would not be a contraindication.

→ http://www.rcog.org.uk/what-we-do/campaigning-and-opinions/briefings-and-qas-/rcog-and-hrt-debate

5. E ★ OHCS 8th edn → p49

Magnesium sulphate is the evidence-based treatment for eclamptic seizures. She also needs her blood pressure controlling carefully and delivery expedited.

→ http://www.rcog.org.uk/womens-health/clinical-guidance/management-severe-pre-eclampsiaeclampsia-green-top-10a

6. B ★   OHCS 8th edn → p48

Although she is currently asymptomatic her blood pressure is >160/100 mmHg and she has significant proteinuria, despite labetalol. She needs admission for careful monitoring and controlled management with antihypertensives, and consideration of delivery if there is no improvement.

7. C ★   OHCS 8th edn → p297

The girl appears Gillick competent as she understands the nature of the treatment; therefore, she should be prescribed emergency contraception like any other patient. Emergency contraception can be given up to 72h after unprotected sex. Thought must be given to ongoing contraception to avoid further incidents.
→ http://www.dh.gov.uk/en/Publichealth/Healthimprovement/ Sexualhealth/Sexualhealthgeneralinformation/DH_4001998

8. B ★   OHCS 8th edn → p284

Hyphae indicate the presence of *Candida* or 'thrush'. Antibiotics are not appropriate treatment for a fungal infection. Clotrimazole is an antifungal topical treatment.

9. A ★   OHCS 8th edn → pp300–302

Most people remember that there is some interaction between the Pill and antibiotics. In truth, the evidence is slight, but the official advice to women taking the combined oral contraceptive pill is to use additional contraceptive methods for the duration of the course and for 7 oral-contraceptive-pill-taking days afterwards (i.e. the pill-free week does not 'count' so if a pill-free week is coming up, she might want to run two packets together).

However, this rule does not apply to progestogen-only contraceptive pills, such as Cerazette®, and she should continue taking it continuously at the same time every day.
→ http://www.nhs.uk/Conditions/Combined-contraceptive-pill/Pages/ Interactions--other-medicines.aspx

10. E ★   OHCS 8th edn → pp54, 62

The reason inductions are booked at 42 weeks is that the risk of intrauterine death increases significantly after this.

11. B ★   EOG → p147; OHCS 8th edn → p84

Massaging the uterus helps to stimulate a contraction; the commonest cause is uterine atony. Syntocinon IM is the first-line treatment. It is a synthetic version of oxytocin and stimulates contractions. If bleeding does not stop, syntocinon infusion and carboprost can be used along with other approaches for a major haemorrhage, such as blood transfusion and fresh frozen plasma. Blood loss of over 1000mL, or clinical signs of shock, are seen as being a major incident.

12. D ★   OHCS 8th edn → p286

A, B, and E are ineffective versus *Chlamydia* and C is contraindicated in pregnancy

13. C ★   OHCS 8th edn → p307

Detrusor contraction is activated via muscarinic cholinergic receptors and oxybutynin is a direct antimuscarinic agent. Serotonin and noradrenaline (norepinephrine) are important for sympathetic activation, which reduces detrusor activity intrinsically. There are no nicotinic or GABAergic receptors in the bladder.

14. A ★

E. coli is by far the commonest cause of sporadic or catheter-related UTI. *Pseudomonas* is usually only associated with prolonged catheterization and *S. epidermidis* is usually a contaminant.

15. B ★   OHCS 8th edn → p284

This is a description of bacterial vaginosis, which is composed of an altered vaginal flora and overgrowth of a number of different micro-organisms, which may show up on Gram staining.

16. D ★   OHCS 8th edn → p50

This woman has gone into premature labour but is at an early stage, so there is a possibility that it can be stopped with tocolytics. However, steroids should still be given to mature the fetal lungs in case delivery goes ahead. There is no indication of infection so antibiotics are not routinely given.
→ http://www.rcog.org.uk/womens-health/clinical-guidance/antenatal-corticosteroids-prevent-respiratory-distress-syndrome-gree

17. B ★

The doctor has to judge whether the girl is Gillick competent, and if she is, then she can consent to treatment herself. However, if she is thought to be the victim of any kind of sexual abuse/coercion, then child protection rules trump her right of confidentiality and the doctor has a duty of care to at least seek advice, for example from the local Child Protection Team. The General Medical Council (GMC) gives guidance on this, which should be read.
→ http://www.gmc-uk.org/guidance/current/library/confidentiality.asp#29

18. B ★   OHCS 8th edn → pp272–273

All of these are protective against cervical changes. HPV vaccination has now been introduced into the UK and will help prevent changes occurring, but in this case, when the changes are already present, it will not be effective. The evidence shows that smoking is the most important risk factor in women who have mild change.

19. C ★

Combined pills are no longer used for post-coital contraception. There is no efficacy advantage, and they have more side effects than Levonelle® (a progestogen-only pill). Levonelle® may be an option. However, it does not offer the additional benefit of an on-going method of contraceptive, and there is also a recognized failure rate. An IUD is always the most effective form of post-coital contraception (for anyone), but in this case it has the added advantage of providing on-going contraception (this is her second condom accident in 2 months and she cannot tolerate oral contraceptives). Mirena® coils are not used for post-coital contraception.

20. A ★

Chlamydia is the commonest sexually transmitted infection in the UK; 50% of men have no symptoms but those that do may have dysuria, epididymo-orchitis, clear penile discharge, and low-grade fever.

21. D ★

Pneumocystis jirovecii (previously known as *Pneumocystis carinii*) can cause severe pneumonia (*Pneumocystis carinii* pneumonia or PCP) in immunocompromised individuals. The risk increases when CD4+ cell numbers fall below 200×10^6/L, especially if viral load is detectable; therefore measures are taken to try and prevent this with antibiotic prophylaxis. It has been standard practice for many years to offer HIV patients with a CD4+ count less than 200 /μl primary prophylaxis against *Pneumocystis*. Without antiviral therapy, *Pneumocystis* is the single most likely serious/life-threatening opportunistic infection they will get. Patients can get *Cryptococcus*, but it is much less common, and primary prophylaxis is not given, although secondary prophylaxis would be continued in those who do get it until their CD4+ count came up in response to antiviral therapy. *M. avium intracellulare* is unlikely to be a problem with a CD4+ count >100 /μl, and primary prophylaxis is not routinely given. *M. tuberculosis* can of course affect any patient regardless of CD4+ count, but primary prophylaxis is not given.

T. gondii is unlikely to be a problem with a CD4+ count >50 /μl so primary prophylaxis would not be given at this CD4+ count.

22. B ★   OHCS 8th edn → p268

Genital herpes causes multiple, painful sores on the vulva, which may also cause lymphadenopathy and flu-like symptoms. Behçet's syndrome can cause genital ulceration but is rare. Lichen sclerosus causes white, atrophic-looking areas and usually occurs in older women. Syphilitic chancres are usually single and ulcerated.

23. B ★ ★   OHCS 8th edn → p268

This is herpes simplex virus infection, so antiviral treatment is required.

24. C ★ ★   OHCS 8th edn → pp44–45

This is a normal CTG, with a baseline of between 110 and 160bpm, a variability of >5bpm, and accelerations seen.

25. B ★ ★

General principles of consent mean that the patient is the only person capable of giving consent for any investigation or treatment. However, if the medical information may guide his treatment, for example deciding which drugs to start, then investigations can be performed when he is unable to give consent. This is rarely straightforward, however, and the GMC guidance on consent should be read. Universal precautions mean that full infection control precautions should be taken for *all* patients, regardless of whether they are known to be HIV positive or not.
→ http://www.gmc-uk.org/guidance/ethical_guidance/consent_guidance/scope_of_treatment_in_emergancies.asp

26. A ★ ★   OHCS 8th edn → p281

Adenomata by definition are derived from the ovarian glandular epithelium.

27. C ★ ★   OHCS 8th edn → p252

A reversed LH:FSH ratio of around 3:1 and numerous small peripheral follicles in the ovaries is characteristic of polycystic ovarian syndrome. The symptoms of this include reduced periods, reduced fertility, hirsutism, acne, and weight gain.

28. C ★ ★

This patient has detectable HBcAb. The only way you get core antibody is by having hepatitis B virus infection. There is no core antigen in the vaccine. However, he is HBsAg negative and HBeAg negative, so he is not a chronic virus carrier. Unfortunately, he has not developed any HBsAb, which is the antibody that conveys protective immunity (and what the vaccine aims to produce). There is some controversy about whether vaccinating patients with a blunted response to prior hepatitis B virus infection does anything (if the infection did not result in immunity, then the vaccine is unlikely to do any better). However, there is no evidence base for it.

29. D ★   OHCS 8th edn → p250

Mefenamic acid is effective for period pain and can be taken around the time of the period only. Tranexamic acid has some pain-relieving properties but is better for heavy periods. An IUS would be an option, but she is not sexually active so this would not be the first-line management. The pill may lighten periods, but does not necessarily help pain. Gonadotrophin-releasing hormone analogues have no role.

30. B ★ ★   OHCS 8th edn → p35

Risks with modern management using antiretrovirals and elective caesarean section are very low, although not eliminated completely.

31. C ★ ★   OHCS 8th edn → p263

Whilst the history and empty uterus here are suggestive of ectopic pregnancy, the β-HCG level is only just <1000mIU/mL. The woman is not shocked, so urgent treatment is not needed. β-HCG normally doubles over 48h, so a repeat test may confirm the diagnosis and allow decisions to about management to be made. If the β-HCG has not doubled, then this is strongly suggestive of an ectopic pregnancy.
→ http://www.rcog.org.uk/files/rcog-corp/uploaded-files/ GT21ManagementTubalPregnancy2004.pdf

32. C ★ ★   OHCS 8th edn → p52

Serial ultrasound scans to detect changes in abdominal circumference are accurate at diagnosing growth restriction. As this baby's abdominal circumference is less than the 10th centile, it may be growth restricted and a scan should be repeated after 2 weeks.
→ http://www.rcog.org.uk/files/rcog-corp/uploaded-files/ GT31SmallGestationalAgeFetus.pdf

33. D ★ ★

If the donor in a needle-stick injury is high risk for blood-borne viruses, then PEP should be started straight away until confirmatory testing can be done. Delays reduce the effectiveness. Many antiretrovirals are safe in pregnancy; indeed, pregnant HIV-positive women are advised to take antiretrovirals to reduce the risk of transmission to the fetus.
→ http://www.nice.org.uk/niceMedia/documents/pep.pdf

34. C ★ ★   OHCS 8th edn → pp10–11

The triple test measures maternal serum levels of α-fetoprotein, human chorionic gonadotrophin and unconjugated oestriol. It uses these levels, along with maternal age, to calculate the risk of certain conditions. It is a screening tool and is not diagnostic. If the risk is high, mothers can choose further diagnostic tests if they wish.

35. A ★★

There are four stages of syphilis:

- Primary: characterized by painless ulcers, called chancres, at the site of infection, which may not be noticed. These occur about 3 weeks after infection.

- Secondary: occurs 2–10 weeks after the chancres and symptoms include a rash, mouth ulcers, lymphadenopathy, fever, and myalgia.

- Latent: occurs months to years after the initial infection if it goes untreated and is usually asymptomatic, but the infection remains in the body.

- Tertiary: occurs years after initial infection in a minority of people and can affect almost any part of the body.

Testing for syphilis can be complex because of the different stages. However, in someone who is asymptomatic but has positive serological tests, this implies the infection is latent. If you *know* the patient acquired the infection within the last 2 years, then it is early latent. In this case, we can be completely confident that the infection is less than 2 years old because we are told that the syphilis serology was negative 18 months ago.

36. A ★★   OHCS 8th edn → p48

These symptoms indicate severe pre-eclampsia. Brisk reflexes are commonly associated with pre-eclampsia. The rest are just general signs.

37. D ★★   OHCS 8th edn → pp262–263

The commonest cause of arrest and death in early pregnancy is hypovolaemia due to ruptured ectopic pregnancy and is the first consideration in a collapsed patient in early pregnancy. Heavy vaginal bleeding rarely presents in arrest, as help tends to be sought early for visible bleeding. The risk of pulmonary embolus is raised throughout pregnancy, but the most severe morbidity and mortality is in later trimesters or post-partum, and both sepsis due to termination and pre-existing cardiac conditions are fortunately rare.
→ http://www.cemach.org.uk/getdoc/0dd34f16-5488-4c85-b9c8-567d44208abe/Chapter6.aspx

38. A ★ ★ ★

Someone with marked tenderness should not be allowed home. The history, examination and ultrasound scan findings are highly suggestive and commensurate with a haemorrhagic cyst accident, which should be managed conservatively. The absence of vomiting, peritonism, and a pyrexia make torsion and appendicitis unlikely, and there is no need to refer to the surgeons at this stage as the diagnosis is basically straightforward. As such, no further imaging is required at this stage.

39. A ★ ★ ★   OHCS 8th edn → p266

This is lichen sclerosus et atrophicus, a poorly understood inflammatory condition. It responds well to potent corticosteroid ointment, and biopsy is indicated if there is no response to treatment or if an actual suspicious lesion such as an ulcer is present. Oestrogen cream works for pure atrophy only and the likelihood of a sexually transmitted infection in a 70 year old is very small. Excision is left for neoplastic conditions.

40. D ★ ★ ★   OHCS 8th edn → p288

All of the medical treatments listed are effective for pain, although there is increasing evidence that surgery has the best results overall. Endometriomata tend to respond poorly to medical treatment and usually need excision. Only surgical treatment has been proven to improve subsequent fertility.

41. C ★ ★ ★

Primary pelvic clearance and tumour debulking are the mainstays of ovarian cancer treatment initially. Neoadjuvant chemotherapy is reasonable in some women, but involves carboplatin and paclitaxel, not vincristine. Hormonal treatment and radiotherapy have little or no place in ovarian cancer treatment, and palliative care is for women with terminal disease who have not responded to surgery and chemotherapy.

42. A ★ ★ ★ ★

Patients who have had a seizure should refrain from driving for 1 year. It is the patient's responsibility to inform the DVLA, who may then seek information from the doctor. However, the doctor should inform patients of this as they may be unaware.
→ http://www.epilepsysociety.org.uk/AboutEpilepsy/ Livingwithepilepsy/Drivingandtravel/Drivingandtransport

Extended Matching Questions

1. I ★

Although testicular pain should always be taken seriously, this young man has bilateral pain associated with fever and possible lymph node and parotid swelling.

This suggests mumps. Although the treatment is supportive, the worry is about subfertility in post-pubertal men following mumps.

2. F ★

In contrast to the previous question, this pain is severe and unilateral. The milder episodes may well have been the testis retracting and twisting slightly in the past, but this severe episode suggests torsion, and he needs emergency surgical exploration to save the testicle.

3. H ★

This is a varicocele – an enlargement of the veins that drain the testicle, the pampiniform plexus. It is similar to varicose veins in the leg. It tends to be more noticeable when standing, in keeping with gravity. It is usually painless, but may be treated surgically if causing problems. There may be a small increased risk of infertility, but most men with these are not infertile.

4. E ★

Chlamydia is the commonest sexually transmitted infection and causes epididymo-orchitis and urethral discharge. Gonorrhoea also causes discharge, but this is usually yellow and slimy, and dysuria is also prominent. Doxycycline or azithromycin are the usual first-line treatments for *Chlamydia*, but a diagnostic urine test should be sent first. Broad-spectrum antibiotics and most penicillins are not routinely used.

5. J ★

A firm, solid, painless testicular lump is a testicular tumour until proven otherwise and should be referred to urology for diagnosis and treatment.

General feedback on 1–5: When assessing testicular problems, differential diagnosis should include: testicular torsion (acute, excruciatingly painful, and tender), which is a surgical emergency; tumour (firm, painless, non-cystic lump); epididymo-orchitis (discomfort and swelling, especially at the back of the scrotum, and possibly some discharge), which is usually caused by a sexually transmitted infection, such as *Chlamydia*, or bacteria that cause UTI. Benign conditions include a varicocele, which does not usually cause any problems.

6. H ★

This is most likely as there are no clinical or ultrasound features of malignancy. The simple nature excludes a dermoid cyst, which is heterogeneous on scan.

7. B ★

This represents a large transformation zone (area of squamous metaplasia), usually due to the high oestrogen levels seen with the combined pill. It is physiological, but may cause post-coital bleeding and therefore concern.

8. M ★

This is commonly ulcerated and on the labia majora. Vulval intraepithelial neoplasia may be white and plaque-like but not ulcerated, and melanoma is usually pigmented.

9. J ★

These are very common and lead to uterine enlargement. If inside the cavity, they can cause heavy periods.

10. E ★

Post-menopausal bleeding is endometrial adenocarcinoma until proven otherwise—her age, obesity, and diabetes are also risk factors for endometrial adenocarcinoma. A normal smear 12 months previously makes cervical carcinoma less likely.

General feedback on 6–10: OHCS 8th edn → pp250, 266, 278

11. K ★

UTI is common in pregnancy and these are typical symptoms.

12. J ★

This is likely to be an ectopic pregnancy, with abdominal pain and cervical excitation in the first trimester of pregnancy. A transvaginal ultrasound scan is the most sensitive way of confirming an empty uterus and looking at the Fallopian tubes to try and identify the pregnancy.

13. B ★

This woman is likely to have a molar pregnancy, or hydatidiform mole. This is a rare occurrence caused by either a placenta only developing with no fetus, or a fetus with too many chromosomes developing with an abnormal placenta. The placenta produces β-HCG in large amounts, so this will indicate the diagnosis. The typical ultrasound appearance is of a 'snow storm' uterus.

14. H ★

Hyperemesis gravidarum is severe morning sickness. Large amounts of vomiting can cause metabolic disturbance and may need to be treated with IV fluids.

15. L ★

The commonest cause of amenorrhea is still pregnancy!

General feedback on 11–15: OHCS 8th edn → pp17, 260, 262

16. N ★

These are classical prolapse symptoms, for which a ring pessary may be a first-line solution. Lack of urinary and bowel symptoms makes anterior or posterior prolapse less likely.

17. D ★

Urgency and incontinence are most likely to represent detrusor overactivity.

18. B ★

Continuous leaking is suggestive of a bladder bypass. The age and presence of a congenital vaginal septum (40% coexistence with urinary abnormalities) suggest a congenital abnormality, e.g. aberrant-ending ureter in vagina.

19. L ★

20–30% of women with *Chlamydia* have symptoms, often urinary. *Chlamydia* infects the anterior urethra and is described as urethritis (not a UTI).

20. F ★

The trigone is oestrogen sensitive and atrophy can lead to urinary symptoms as well as vulvo-vaginal symptoms. A good response to local oestrogen cream is characteristic.

General feedback on 15–20: OHCS 8th edn → pp306–307

21. F ★

Gestational diabetes can go unrecognized and leads to macrosomia and a large-for-dates baby, which can cause problems in vaginal delivery.

22. L ★

This is hypertension in pregnancy plus proteinuria, often with peripheral oedema. It can be asymptomatic, hence the need for blood pressure monitoring in pregnancy. However, headache and abdominal pain are symptoms that require further investigation and management.

23. M ★

Risk for pulmonary embolism is raised in pregnancy. Other risk factors here are the unexpected immobility. Pulmonary embolism causes pleuritic chest pain, shortness of breath, tachycardia, and hypoxia. It can be fatal so needs to be recognized and treated.

24. H ★

Anaemia is common in pregnancy because of the increased demand by the fetus and haemodilution by the increased plasma volume. Not all women need treatment; the World Health Organization (WHO) advises keeping levels above 11g/dL. However, this woman has a markedly decreased Hb level and symptoms of anaemia, namely tiredness. Her MCV and MCHC are low, indicating iron deficiency.

25. C ★

If left untreated, pre-eclampsia can progress and cause seizures. This is eclampsia. The low blood pressure here is post-ictal.

General feedback on 21–25: OHCS 8th edn → pp22, 24, 32, 48

CHAPTER 2
PAEDIATRICS

Jennifer Birch, Johnathan Darling, Luci Etheridge, and Matthew Mathai

Children are not merely small adults. To be a good paediatrician requires as much knowledge about health as about disease. The normal patterns of growth and development can be a mystery to many, and paediatricians are often called upon to help interpret these for confused parents. There is a unique need to be aware of the range of congenital disorders that may present before, at, or shortly after birth. Younger children cannot tell us their symptoms; paediatricians have to learn to pick up on non-verbal clues and often subtle signs when the answer may lie in something unexpected and far removed from the traditional history and examination format. At the other end of the spectrum, adolescents have their own range of health issues and are traditionally an under-represented and often forgotten group. In this chapter, we aim to cover many of the key presentations and issues in children of all ages, from neonates to teenagers.

Even in this modern age, children are susceptible to infection. Respiratory and gastrointestinal infections are the commonest presentations in both general practice and paediatric hospital practice. Fortunately, most of these infections are self-limiting, but serious infections do occur and must be recognized. However, the leading cause of death in all children over 1 year of age is accidents. Recognizing risk factors for accidental and non-accidental harm is a major responsibility for all those working with children.

The questions in this chapter will test the common areas that present to paediatricians but also relevant issues such as knowledge of disease factors, ethics, and risk management in relation to children and their families. The best way, however, to learn about children is to get out there and meet them: play with them, talk to parents and carers, and see them when they are ill and well. You will learn the most this way and be able to apply that knowledge and experience to answer questions such as these. ∎

Luci Etheridge

SINGLE BEST ANSWERS

1. A 1-day-old girl has a harsh systolic cardiac murmur all over the precordium with a thrill at the left sternal edge. Femoral pulses are palpable. A chest X-ray shows an enlarged heart and an ECG shows left ventricular hypertrophy. Which is the single most likely diagnosis? ★

A Aortic stenosis

B Coarctation of the aorta

C Patent ductus arteriosus

D Pulmonary stenosis

E Ventricular septal defect

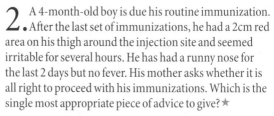

2. A 4-month-old boy is due his routine immunization. After the last set of immunizations, he had a 2cm red area on his thigh around the injection site and seemed irritable for several hours. He has had a runny nose for the last 2 days but no fever. His mother asks whether it is all right to proceed with his immunizations. Which is the single most appropriate piece of advice to give? ★

A Immunization should be postponed until his runny nose has settled

B Immunize him in hospital

C Omit pertussis but proceed with other immunizations

D Omit this set of immunizations

E Reassure and proceed with planned immunizations now

3. A 7-year-old girl is drowsy and panting and has a capillary blood glucose of 25mmol/L and ketones and protein in her urine. Initial blood results show:

- Sodium 145mmol/L
- Potassium 3.8mmol/L
- Creatinine 100µmol/L
- Urea 12mmol/L
- Calcium 2.6mmol/L
- Glucose 26mmol/L

She is given two fluid boluses of 10ml/kg 0.9% saline and is then started on a 0.9% saline infusion to deliver a total of maintenance plus 10% over 48h IV insulin is also started. Two hours later she has improved, has passed urine, and is more alert. Her blood results show:

- Sodium 143mmol/L
- Potassium 3.8mmol/L
- Creatinine 82µmol/L
- Urea 10mmol/L
- Calcium 2.2mmol/L
- Glucose 20mmol/L

Which single fluid should she now be given intravenously? ★

A 0.45% saline and 5% dextrose

B 0.45% saline and 5% dextrose with added calcium

C 0.45% saline and 5% dextrose with added potassium

D 0.9 % saline

E 0.9% saline with added potassium

4. A 5-year-old girl had been passing hard stools once every 5–7 days for 6 months. She was started on two Movicol® Paediatric sachets daily. She took this for 1 month and she started passing a stool every day, so her parents stopped it. For the last month, she has been soiling her pants, with intermittent runny stools. She opens her bowels on the toilet most days and passes pellet-like stools and an occasional large, hard stool. Which is the single main deficiency in her management so far? ★

A Colonoscopy should have been performed

B Glycerol suppositories should have been added

C Movicol® should have been continued for several more months

D She should have had an enema when first seen

E Stimulant laxatives should have been used

5. A 7-year-old boy wets the bed most nights and has never been reliably dry. He is a heavy sleeper. He has kept a star chart for 4 weeks and his parents have been supportive. His chart shows one dry night each week, with no particular pattern. He has a cub camp in 4 months' time. Urinalysis is negative. Which is the single most appropriate management? ★

A Star chart

B Enuresis alarm

C Desmopressin melts at night

D Imipramine tablets at night

E Oxybutynin tablets at night

6. A 1-year-old boy has had diarrhoea for the past 12h. At the beginning of the illness, he vomited twice. He has not passed urine for the past 6h. He is thirsty and restless, his eyes are sunken, the mucous membranes are dry, and skin turgor has decreased. His pulse rate is 160bpm. His capillary refill time is 2 s. Which is the single best description of his degree of dehydration and the appropriate initial fluid to give? ★

A Mild; oral rehydration solution

B Mild; 0.9% saline IV

C Moderate; oral rehydration solution

D Moderate; 0.9% saline IV

E Severe; 0.9% saline IV

7. A 20-hour-old term newborn boy has a short, soft, early systolic murmur on his baby check. He is pink, with no signs of respiratory distress, and has normally palpable femoral pulses and a normal apex beat. The murmur is heard at the upper left sternal edge, radiates through the chest, and there are no associated heaves or thrills. Which is the single most likely diagnosis? ★

A Atrial septal defect

B Innocent heart murmur

C Patent ductus arteriosus

D Pulmonary stenosis

E Ventricular septal defect

8. A 12-year-old girl, recently arrived in the UK from South Asia, has had pain and swelling of both knees, ankles, and wrists for 5 days, which comes and goes. Five weeks ago, she had a cold and sore throat. For the last day, she has had a rash on her trunk, which has a pink border and is fading centrally. Both knees have an effusion and limited flexion to 70°. Her temperature is 39.2°C and her pulse rate is 160bpm. Which single organism is likely to be responsible for this illness? ★

A *Corynebacterium diphtheriae*

B Human cytomegalovirus

C Epstein–Barr virus

D Group A β-haemolytic *Streptococcus*

E *Staphylococcus aureus*

9. A 6-year-old boy has had vomiting for 24h and has been unable to keep any liquids down, although he hasn't wanted to eat any food. Today he has central abdominal pain, which was coming and going but is now constant and sharp. He has pain when he tries to pass urine and gets very upset if he is moved. He has opened his bowels once today and passed a loose stool. Which is the single most likely diagnosis? ★

A Appendicitis

B Gastro-oesophageal reflux

C Mesenteric adenitis

D Viral gastroenteritis

E Volvulus

10. A 39-week, 3.4kg baby girl is due her baby check. The baby is lying supine. The examiner's left hand is stabilizing the pelvis and his right hand is grasping the left leg, flexed at the hip and knee, with his thumb over the lesser trochanter and the tip of his middle finger over the greater trochanter. The examiner wants first to check if the right hip is dislocatable with Barlow's manoeuvre. Which is the single most accurate description of how the examination should be performed? ★

A Adduct the leg to the midline and apply gentle anterior pressure over the greater trochanter

B Adduct the leg to the midline and apply gentle posterior pressure over the lesser trochanter

C Fully abduct the leg and apply gentle posterior pressure over the lesser trochanter

D Fully abduct the leg and apply gentle anterior pressure over the greater trochanter

E Partially abduct the leg and apply gentle anterior pressure over the greater trochanter

11. A 24-month-old girl enjoys 'feeding' her dolls. She does not like taking turns. She is able to walk upstairs with help but is unable to stand on one leg. She is able to scribble but is unable to draw a circle. She can say 'mama' and 'dada' with meaning but no other recognizable words. In which single developmental area is she showing delay? ★

A Fine motor skills

B Gross motor skills

C Social skills

D Speech and language skills

E Play skills

12. A 14-year-old girl has chronic kidney disease. Her nephrologist advises that dialysis is the only option while awaiting renal transplant. She refuses to have dialysis and appears to understand the consequence of not having treatment. She had been in and out of local authority care between the age of 1 and 6 years, but has been back with her parents for the last 8 years. Her mother, who holds sole parental responsibility, wants her to have dialysis, but her father feels that she should decide for herself. The family have been through extensive counselling with the team, but have not been able to reach a consensus. Which single decision takes precedence when deciding further management? ★

A The father's

B The local authority's

C The mother's

D The nephrologist's

E The patient's

13. A 2-month-old boy has faltering growth. He is a sweaty baby, particularly on breastfeeding. He has a palpable 4cm liver edge. He is pale and has a respiratory rate of 60/min, a heart rate of 180bpm, a blood pressure of 80/40mmHg, and his oxygen saturation is 96% in air. His capillary refill time is 3s. Capillary blood glucose is 5mmol/L. Which single system of the body is most likely to be affected? ★

A Cardiovascular system

B Gastrointestinal system

C Metabolic system

D Neurological system

E Respiratory system

14. A 37-week baby weighing 2.7kg at birth is now 4 days old. He is breastfed. During the first 24h of life, he did not latch on to the breast well and fed for approximately 5min at a time every 4–5h. He is now feeding for 15–20min every 2–3h. His weight today is 2.55kg. His mother is worried about his weight loss. Which is the single most appropriate advice to give her? ★

A Any weight loss in the first week is worrying and he should have supplementary feeds

B He has lost less than 10% of his birth weight, which is acceptable in the first week, and she should continue breastfeeding

C He has lost less than 10% of his birth weight, which is acceptable in the first week, but he should have supplementary feeds until he gains weight

D He has lost more than 10% of his birth weight, which is acceptable in the first week, and she should continue breastfeeding

E He has lost more than 10% of his birth weight, which is more than is normal in the first week, so he should have supplementary feeds

15. A 14-year-old Caucasian boy has had temperatures with drenching night sweats and malaise for 8 weeks. He has lost 4kg in weight. He had a venticular septal defect repaired in infancy. He looks pale, has extensive dental decay, and small, linear areas of bleeding under his nail beds. He has a three-finger-breadth splenomegaly and a grade 2 systolic murmur heard best in the lower left sternal edge. His temperature is 38°C. Which is the single most appropriate treatment? ★

A Antibiotics

B Chemotherapy

C Diuretics

D High-dose steroids

E Surgery

16. An 18-month-old African-Caribbean girl is not yet walking. She was breastfed for 9 months and is thriving along the 25th centile for weight. She has bow legs, Harrison's sulci, and swollen wrists. Which single vitamin deficiency is she most likely to have? ★

A Vitamin A

B Vitamin B$_{12}$

C Vitamin C

D Vitamin D

E Vitamin E

17. A mother brings her 7-month-old boy to the Emergency Department. She says he is always on the go and that morning she saw him climb out of his cot and fall onto laminate flooring, from a height of approximately 3 feet. He is now not moving his right leg. He has a spiral fracture of the right femur on X-ray. Which single part of the history will help most in deciding further management? ★

A Birth history

B Family medical history

C Developmental history

D Social history

E Systems review questioning

18. A 4-year-old Caucasian boy has poorly controlled asthma, despite being on a high-dose steroid inhaler and a leukotriene receptor antagonist and compliant with his medication. He has recurrent chest infections and has significant nasal discharge. He has poor growth, Harrison's sulci, and finger clubbing. Which is the single most appropriate next investigation? ★

A Bronchial brush biopsy

B Bronchoalveolar lavage

C CT scan of the chest

D Lung function tests

E Sweat test

19. A 4-year-old boy has periorbital oedema, central abdominal discomfort, and decreased urine output. His urine dipstick shows 3+ proteinuria and no blood. He is asthmatic and recently had a bad 'cold'. Which is the single most likely diagnosis? ★

A Angioedema

B Nephrotic syndrome

C Post-streptococcal glomerulonephritis

D Postural proteinuria

E Systemic lupus erythematosis (SLE)

20. A 7-year-old boy with asthma has had a 'cold' and a temperature of 37.7°C for 24h. He has severe respiratory distress and requires 15L/min of oxygen to maintain his oxygen saturation over 95%. He is started on nebulized salbutamol therapy, which causes an initial improvement in his symptoms. He then suddenly deteriorates, with marked respiratory distress, hypoxia, and hypotension. Which is the single most likely diagnosis? ★

A Anaphylaxis

B Pleural effusion

C Pneumonia

D Pulmonary embolus

E Tension pneumothorax

$\left(21.\right)$ A 6-year-old girl has had vomiting and central abdominal pain for 3 days. She has eczema and poorly controlled asthma. She looks pale and has a Glasgow Coma Scale score of 11/15. Her abdomen is generally tender, but there is no rigidity, rebound, or guarding. Bowel sounds are present and normal. Her respiratory rate is 36/min, with no recession. Her heart rate is 160bpm and capillary refill time is 4s. She is given a 20mL/kg bolus of fluid. Blood tests show:

- Haemoglobin 13g/dL
- White cell count 22 × 10⁹/L
- C-reactive protein 25mg/L
- Sodium 120mmol/L
- Potassium 6.8mmol/L
- Urea 9.3mmol/L
- Creatinine 110µmol/L

Which is the single most important next investigation? ★

A Abdominal ultrasound scan

B Blood glucose

C CT scan of the head

D Serum ammonia

E Urine osmolality

22. A 3-year-old boy is in acute respiratory distress. There is no past history of note except that he has not been immunized. He has a temperature of 40°C, looks flushed and unwell, is drooling, and has an inspiratory stridor. His cough is muffled. A colleague asks for help examining the boy's throat. Which is the single most appropriate advice to give? ★

A Do not disturb the child and call for senior help urgently

B Give nebulized budesonide and then examine the throat

C Go ahead and examine the throat, but have a laryngoscope and endotracheal tube to hand

D Go ahead and examine the throat straight away to help make a diagnosis

E Site an intravenous line and give a dose of cefotaxime first, and then examine the throat

23. A 9-month-old boy has had a generalized seizure, lasting 5min, where he stared straight ahead and his arms and legs shook. He had been unwell for 12h with fever, runny nose, and cough. He has never had any fits before and there is no family history of epilepsy. His development had been appropriate for age, but in the last 6 weeks he has stopped pulling to stand or cruising round furniture. His temperature is 39°C and he has pharyngitis. A diagnosis of febrile convulsion is made. Which single feature in the history is least consistent with a diagnosis of febrile convulsion? ★

A Absence of previous febrile fits

B Age of child

C Description of seizure

D Developmental history

E Duration of seizure

24. A 3-month-old baby girl has dry skin on her scalp, as shown in Plate 2.1. It has been present for the past 5 weeks and is getting progressively worse. Which is the single most likely diagnosis? ★

A Atopic eczema

B Impetigo

C Psoriasis

D Seborrhoeic dermatitis

E Tinea capitis

25. A 2.8kg, 37-week baby girl has been treated briefly with phototherapy for jaundice. She is now 7 days old, breastfeeding well, and starting to regain weight. She has been off phototherapy for over 48h and her bilirubin chart is shown in Plate 2.2. Her mother has heard someone mention that her baby has 'breast milk jaundice' and wants to know how she should continue to feed her baby. Which is the single most appropriate advice to give the mother? ★ ★

A She should continue to breastfeed but also give some extra formula feeds to ensure a good milk intake to help reduce the jaundice

B She should continue to breastfeed exclusively as it is still the best milk for her baby, regardless of the jaundice, which is already improving

C She should give mainly formula milk for the next 3 weeks with the occasional breastfeed to ensure an ongoing breast milk supply

D She should stop breastfeeding completely and change to a term formula to prevent the jaundice from worsening again

E She should stop breastfeeding for 48h to allow the jaundice level to fall further and then restart

26. A 12-year-old girl has short stature. She had a birth weight of 2kg at term and had a coarctation of the aorta repair in infancy. She has bilateral ptosis, a low posterior hairline and multiple pigmented naevi. She plots on the 0.4th centile for height and 2nd centile for weight. Her mid-parental height centile is the 50th centile. Which single investigation is most likely to lead to a diagnosis? ★ ★

A Chest X-ray

B Coeliac screen

C Follicle-stimulating hormone and luteinizing hormone levels

D Karyotype

E MRI scan of brain

27. A 20-month-old South Asian boy has bow legs. He was breastfed until 6 months of age. The family live in a 6th floor, two-bedroom flat and his mother wears the hijab. He has mild genu varum bilaterally. His wrist X-ray is shown in Plate 2.3. Which single area of the X-ray shows the bony abnormalities that indicate the likely diagnosis? ★ ★

A Carpal bones

B Diaphyses of long bones

C Epiphyses of long bones

D Metacarpal bones

E Metaphyses of long bones

28. A 6-hour-old term baby boy weighs 2.54kg. He has microcephaly, a flat occiput, upwards-slanting palpebral fissures, a protruding tongue, a single palmar crease on the right hand but normal palmar creasing on the left, and a wide sandal gap. Which is the single most likely finding on neurological examination? ★ ★

A Absent Moro reflex

B Exaggerated Moro reflex

C Generalized hypertonia

D Generalized hypotonia

E Selective hypertonia of the lower limbs

29. A 7-year-old girl has had general malaise and pallor for the past 3 days. She is passing small amounts of urine infrequently. She was unwell the previous week with bloody diarrhoea, but this has now settled. Blood results show:

- Haemoglobin 8.2g/dL
- Platelets 400 × 10⁹/L
- White cell count 10.4 × 10⁹/L
- Sodium 135mmol/L
- Potassium 4.2mmol/L
- Urea 22mmo/L
- Creatinine 230μmol/L
- C-reactive protein 11mg/L

Which single organism is the most likely cause of her illness? ★ ★

A *Clostridium difficile*

B *Escherichia coli*

C *Salmonella typhi*

D *Shigella sonnei*

E *Streptococcus pneumoniae*

30. An 8-year-old boy has had headaches for 12 months. They are usually left-sided and throbbing and are made worse by noise and light. They last for around 12h, during which time he is nauseous but does not vomit. There are no obvious triggers. Paracetamol during attacks is of some benefit. He has one bad attack every 3 weeks on average, missing 1–2 days of school each time. Which is the single most appropriate next step in management? ★ ★

A Anti-emetic during attacks

B CT scan of the head

C Oral pizotifen

D Psychology referral

E Sumatriptan nasal spray

31. A 15-year-old boy is worried that he is shorter than all his friends and that he has not yet started puberty. He is otherwise well. His father started puberty at around the age of 14. His parental heights are both on the 25th centile. His growth chart is shown in Plate 2.4. Which single aspect of his growth and pubertal development will be most likely to assist with diagnosis? ★ ★

A Axillary hair stage

B Height centile

C Height velocity centile

D Pubic hair stage

E Testicular size

32. A 25-week-gestation infant has just been delivered by spontaneous vaginal delivery. The full neonatal resuscitation team is present and the Resuscitaire® has been pre-warmed. The baby is handed to the team and they have started the clock. Which is the single most important action to take next? ★ ★ ★

A Assess the baby's initial Apgar score

B Dry the baby thoroughly and check the heart rate

C Intubate immediately and start ventilation breaths

D Put a hat on the baby's head and a plastic bag over his body

E Suction the mouth under direct vision using a laryngoscope

33. A 14-year-old girl has an osteosarcoma of her tibia. She has worsening pain in her leg. She is on regular oral paracetamol and ibuprofen. Which is the single most appropriate next treatment? ★ ★ ★

A Codeine phosphate

B Diazepam

C Diclofenac

D Hyoscine bromide

E Morphine sulphate

34. A newborn baby boy has a urethral meatus that comes out on the dorsum of the penis, shown in Plate 2.5. He is able to pass a good stream of urine. Which single piece of advice should be given to his parents before discharge? ★ ★ ★

A He should not be circumcised

B He should not wear disposable nappies

C The foreskin should be retracted gently every day

D The penis should be cleaned with mild soapy water daily

E This is entirely normal and nothing further is needed

35. A 4-year-old boy was accidentally given IV cefuroxime 30min ago that was prescribed on the wrong drug chart. He has no relevant allergies and does not seem to have suffered any ill effects. The antibiotic has been crossed off his chart. His parents have now returned to the ward after being at home. Which is the single most appropriate course of action? ★ ★ ★

A Discuss at handover later in the day and write a reflective portfolio entry

B Do nothing further until after discussion with a medical defence organization

C Explain and apologize to the parents and notify a senior colleague promptly

D Notify a senior colleague with a view to explaining the error to the parents later in the day

E Shred the incorrect prescription chart and write a new one before anyone else sees it

36. A 4-month-old girl has been irritable, with a temperature of 38°C for 2 days. She is diagnosed with a coliform urinary tract infection (UTI). Blood and cerebrospinal fluid cultures are negative. She responds to oral anibiotics and is afebrile after 24h. Which single set of investigations should be performed? ★ ★ ★

	Ultrasound of kidneys, ureters, and bladder	Dimercaptosuc-cinic acid (DMSA) renal isotope scan	Micturating cystourethrogram
A	No	No	No
B	Yes	No	No
C	Yes	Yes	No
D	Yes	No	Yes
E	Yes	Yes	Yes

37. A 14-year-old South Asian girl has had polyuria and polydipsia for 4 months. She has a body mass index of 28kg/m² and dark, velvety pigmentation of the skin in her axillae. She has a random serum glucose of 12mmol/L and no blood ketones. Which is the single most likely diagnosis? ★ ★ ★

A Cushing's syndrome

B Diabetes insipidus

C Simple obesity

D Type 1 diabetes mellitus

E Type 2 diabetes mellitus

38. A 30-week-gestation infant is now 12h old. She was in good condition at birth and did not require resuscitation, although she did have some mild subcostal recession and needed 25% incubator oxygen. Over the past few hours, she has developed increasing respiratory distress with grunting, intercostal and subcostal recession, and an increasing oxygen requirement to 45%. Her blood gas shows a respiratory acidosis and her chest X-ray has a homogeneous ground-glass appearance with air bronchograms. She has just been intubated. Which is the single most appropriate medication to give immediately? ★ ★ ★

A Amoxicillin IV

B Dexamethasone IV

C Gentamicin IV

D Morphine infusion IV

E Surfactant via an endotracheal tube

39. A 6-year-old boy is 'always on the go' and finds it difficult to take turns. He is easily distracted and finds it difficult to stick to any task. His father says that he has no sense of danger and often runs across the main road without any care. He has difficulty following a series of simple instructions and is 1 year behind his peers in his numeracy and literacy skills. Which is the single most likely diagnosis? ★ ★ ★

A Attention deficit hyperactivity disorder (ADHD)

B Autism

C Dyspraxia

D Global developmental delay

E Oppositional defiant disorder

40. A 38-week-gestation, 3.1kg baby is delivered by spontaneous vaginal delivery. The pregnancy has been complicated by polyhydramnios. At birth, there are copious oral secretions and respiratory distress. The baby requires intubation and ventilation for respiratory distress and continues to drool. It is not possible to pass a nasogastric tube to the estimated length required and no acid reaction is obtained. Chest X-ray shows the nasogastric tube coiled in the oesophagus, a moderately large stomach bubble, and a normal gas pattern in the bowel. Which is the single most likely diagnosis? ★ ★ ★ ★

A H-type tracheo-oesophageal fistula

B Isolated oesophageal atresia

C Oesophageal atresia and tracheo-oesophageal fistula

D Oesophageal stenosis

E Oesophageal stricture

41. An 8-year-old boy had a throat infection and was given penicillin 2 days ago. He now has a red rash on his trunk, which is peeling, sore red eyes, and has developed lesions on his mouth, shown in Plate 2.6. He looks unwell, has a temperature of 39°C and a heart rate of 175bpm. Which is the single most likely diagnosis? ★ ★ ★ ★

A Bullous impetigo

B Chicken pox

C Hand, foot and mouth disease

D Measles

E Stevens–Johnson syndrome

42. A 9-week-old girl has had brief seizures for the last day, where she stares straight ahead, her body shakes for a few seconds, and her right hand twitches. Pregnancy was normal but delivery was difficult due to shoulder dystocia. Her Apgar scores were 7 at 1min and 9 at 5min. She has some pale areas of skin over her right thigh. She is afebrile. Urea and electrolytes, calcium, magnesium, and glucose are all normal. Lumbar puncture is bloodstained, with a protein of 0.97g/L (normal range up to 0.4g/L). Her electroencephalogram (EEG) is normal. Her MRI brain scan is shown in Plate 2.7. Which is the single most likely diagnosis? ★ ★ ★ ★

A Benign neonatal seizures

B Hypoxic–ischaemic birth injury

C Infantile spasms

D Subdural haematoma

E Tuberous sclerosis

43. Five boys attend the same nursery; are all age 2 years 0 months and, by chance, they all have the same weight of 12.5kg (50th centile). Their parents compare their birth weights and gestations, which are listed as A–E below. Which single child is most at risk of later obesity? ★ ★ ★ ★

	Birth weight (centile)	Gestation (weeks)
A	1.5kg (<0.4th)	40
B	1.5kg (50th)	30
C	2.0kg (98th)	30
D	3.5kg (50th)	40
E	5.0kg (99.6th)	40

44. A 48-hour-old, 2.8kg term baby girl has pallor, poor perfusion, cyanosis, and respiratory distress. She was born in good condition and was well for the first few hours of life. She has been intubated and ventilated, but her oxygen saturations remain between 70 and 80%, despite 100% oxygen and good chest movement. Her femoral pulses are not palpable. Which is the single most appropriate medication to commence next? ★ ★ ★ ★

A Dobutamine

B Dopamine

C Indometacin

D Prostaglandin E_2

E Surfactant

45. A 4-year-old boy has had generalized oedema for 2 days and has 3+ proteinuria on dipstick testing of his urine. His blood pressure is 73/36mmHg. His plasma albumin is 18g/L. All other blood tests, including his urea and electrolytes, are normal. He is started on high-dose daily oral prednisolone. Which single likelihood is there that he will respond to the treatment and not have any further relapses? ★ ★ ★ ★

A 3%

B 30%

C 50%

D 70%

E 90%

EXTENDED MATCHING QUESTIONS

Causes of post-natal ward probelms

For each baby with the clinical sign found on the baby check at approximately 36h old, choose the *single* most likely diagnosis from the list of options below. Each option may be used once, more than once, or not at all. ★

A Benign pustular melanosis

B Candidiasis

C Congenital melanocytic naevus

D Cutis marmorata

E Epstein pearls

F Erythema toxicum neonatorum

G Milia

H Mongolian blue spot

I Neonatal herpes simplex virus

J Port-wine stain

K Stork mark

L Strawberry naevus

1. A 3.2kg term baby has a raised, non-tender, well-demarcated, bright red 0.5cm diameter lesion on his right cheek.

2. A 2.9kg 37-week-gestation baby has 4 small, 1–3mm diameter, white cystic-looking nodules along the midline of the palate.

3. A 4.2kg 41-week-gestation baby has a widespread maculopapular rash with 1–3mm cream papules on an erythematous macular base. The mother reports that the spots seem to 'come and go'.

4. A 3.6kg 39-week-gestation baby has a macular, pink patch over the centre of the neck, forming a roughly triangular shape spreading out slightly towards the hairline.

5. A 3.4kg South Asian baby has a large, blue-black macular discolouration approximately 5cm in diameter over the base of the spine.

?

Causes of abdominal pain

For each child with abdominal pain, choose the *single* most likely diagnosis from the list of options below. Each option may be used once, more than once, or not at all. ★

A Coeliac disease

B Constipation

C Crohn's disease

D Gastroenteritis

E Henoch–Schönlein purpura

F Intussusception

G Lactose intolerance

H Mesenteric adenitis

I Migraine

J Non-organic recurrent abdominal pain

K Pneumonia

L Pyelonephritis

6. A 4-year-old boy has had central abdominal pain for 2 days. He has a palpable purpuric rash on his buttocks and his ankles are swollen.

7. An 8-year-old girl has had lethargy, poor appetite, some weight loss, and right-sided abdominal pain for 5 months. Her stools tend to be loose. Her serum C-reactive protein is 50mg/L.

8. A 15-month-old boy has had sudden bouts of abdominal pain for 12h, when he screams inconsolably, draws his legs up, and becomes very pale. He has passed some reddish, jelly-like stool.

9. An 8-year-old girl has had intermittent, central abdominal pain on and off for 2 years. It lasts for a few minutes, during which she is pale. She has a normal bowel habit. She is growing along the 50th centile.

10. A 3-year-old girl has had poor growth since 9 months of age. Her weight and height are just below the 0.4th centile. She has recurrent abdominal pain and her stools are loose, pale, and difficult to flush. She has a distended abdomen.

Causes of cough

For each child with a cough, choose the *single* most likely diagnosis from the list of options below. Each option may be used once, more than once, or not at all. ★

A Anaphylaxis

B Bacterial tracheitis

C Cystic fibrosis

D Croup

E Epiglottitis

F Foreign body inhalation

G Gastro-oesophageal reflux disease

H Laryngomalacia

I Pertussis

J Tracheo-oesophageal fistula

11. A 14-month-old girl has had a cold for 2 days. She has a hoarse, barking cough and stridor at rest. Her temperature is 37.5°C and she has moderate respiratory distress.

12. A 3-month-old boy has had a cold and worsening cough for 1 week. When he coughs, he goes blue. He has subconjunctival haemorrhages. His blood tests show a white cell count of 26×10^9/L, with neutrophils of 5.5×10^9/L and lymphocytes of 19×10^9/L.

13. A 4-year-old boy is on stage 4 of the British Thoracic Society guidelines for asthma. He is compliant with his medication. He is asymptomatic during the day, but has significant nocturnal cough and wheeze. In the mornings, he has 'really bad breath' and a hoarse voice. There is no family history of atopy. Immunoglobulin E (IgE) levels are normal and tests for house dust mite and other common household allergens are negative.

14. A 1-day-old girl has large amounts of frothy mucus coming out of her mouth and nose. During her first feed, she started coughing and went blue. There was polyhydramnios during the pregnancy.

15. An 18-month-old boy suddenly starts coughing and goes blue, with severe respiratory distress. He has moderate stridor and unilateral wheeze over the left lung, with normal air entry over the right lung.

Causes of floppiness in infants

For each of the following floppy infants, choose the *single* most likely diagnosis from the list below. Each option may be used once, more than once, or not at all. ★

A Congenital myotonic dystrophy

B Central nervous system malformation

C Down's syndrome

D Drug related

E Hypoglycaemia

F Hypothyroidism

G Hypoxic–ischaemic encephalopathy

H Inborn error of metabolism

I Myasthenia gravis

J Prader–Willi syndrome

K Prematurity

L Sepsis

M Spinal muscular atrophy

16. A 2-day-old boy born at 37 weeks' gestation has become jaundiced and floppy and has gone off his feeds in the last 6h. He was breastfeeding well until this point. His mother's membranes ruptured 36h before delivery.

17. A 2-day-old boy born at 38 weeks' gestation has been floppy and feeding poorly since birth. He has a harsh systolic cardiac murmur, loudest at the left sternal edge. He has tiny white speckles on his irises.

18. A 2-day-old boy born at 37 weeks' gestation has had surgery for exomphalos. He has macroglossia and earlobe creases. He is bottle-feeding and has become floppy and pale over the past hour.

19. A 2-day-old girl has been floppy since birth and has just had a 2-second generalized convulsion. She was born by emergency caesarean section for acute placental abruption. Apgar scores were 1 at 1min, 3 at 5min, and 4 at 10min.

20. A 2-day-old South Asian boy born at 37 weeks' gestation has been floppy since 12h of age. His parents are consanguineous. His capillary blood glucose is 3.2mmol/L and capillary pH is 7.1.

Causes of diarrhoea

For each patient with diarrhoea, choose the *single* most likely diagnosis from the list of options below. Each option may be used once, more than once, or not at all. ★

A Coeliac disease

B Cow's milk protein allergy

C Cystic fibrosis

D Galactosaemia

E Infectious enteritis

F Inflammatory bowel disease

G Intussusception

H Poor intake

I Sepsis

J Temporary lactose intolerance

21. A 7-day old breastfed baby has lost 10% of her birth weight. She is lethargic and has a heart rate of 180bpm and a capillary refill time of 4s. Her temperature is 35°C. She has loose, watery stools. Her capillary blood glucose is 3.6mmol/L, serum sodium 132mmol/L, potassium 5mmol/L, urea 8mmol/L, creatinine 70μmol/L, bicarbonate 13mmol/L and C-reactive protein 60mg/L.

22. A 6-year-old boy has had abdominal pain and bloody diarrhoea for 6 months. He has dropped 2 centiles in weight. His abdomen is generally tender. His full blood count shows haemoglobin 8.2g/dL, mean corpuscular volume 79 fL, white cell count 18×10^9/L, and platelets 500×10^9/L.

23. A 6-month-old girl has vomiting, bloody diarrhoea, and abdominal distension, plus widespread eczema. She recently changed from breast milk to formula feeds.

24. A 10-year-old boy with type 1 diabetes has recurrent abdominal pain, oily loose stools, and recurrent episodes of hypoglycaemia.

25. A 3-month-old boy has had severe gastroenteritis, for which he has required intravenous rehydration. On reintroduction of feeds, his diarrhoea has worsened and he has increasing abdominal discomfort and distension and borborygmi.

Causes of limping in children

For each child with difficulty walking, choose the *single* most likely diagnosis from the list of options below. Each option may be used once, more than once, or not at all. ★

A Cerebral palsy

B Developmental dysplasia of the hip

C Henoch–Schönlein purpura

D Idiopathic thrombocytopaenic purpura

E Leukaemia

F Muscular dystrophy

G Myotonic dystrophy

H Perthes' disease

I Slipped upper femoral epiphyses

J Wilson's disease

26. A 3-year-old boy sat independently at 8 months, stood at 16 months, and now has frequent falls and has difficulty climbing stairs. He cannot jump when asked. He walks with short steps and sways his body from side to side.

27. A 2-year-old girl was born at 25 weeks' gestation. She sat at 12 months and stood at 18 months. She has increased tone and reflexes in her legs compared with her arms. When she walks, she is on tiptoe and adducts her legs. Both her upper limbs flex when she walks.

28. A 6-year-old boy has had right-sided hip, groin, and intermittent knee pain for a week. He has limited internal rotation and abduction at the hip, and walks with a limp. There is no history of trauma and no recent illness. He is otherwise well. A full blood count and inflammatory markers are normal.

29. A 14-year-old boy is unsteady on his feet. He has become increasingly aggressive and has slurred speech. He has hepatosplenomegaly, a tremor at rest, and slowed movements.

30. A 4-year-old boy has been limping for 2 days. He has swelling over his left knee joint. He has a palpable purpuric rash on his buttocks. He had a cold a month ago.

Causes of decreased consciousness

For each child with a decreased conscious level, choose the *single* most likely diagnosis from the list of options below. Each option may be used once, more than once, or not at all. ★

A Cerebral oedema

B Encephalitis

C Metabolic defect

D Hypoxia

E Meningitis

F Migraine

G Non-convulsive status epilepticus

H Poisoning

I Stroke

J Wilson's disease

31. A 12-year-old boy has been generally unwell and has had a temperature for 10 days. Over the last 5 days, he has developed a widespread, pruritic rash with erythematous papules, vesicles, and pustules, and some lesions are beginning to crust over. He is drowsy and confused and flexes to pain. There is no focal neurology. His capillary blood glucose is 6mmol/L.

32. A 6-month-old girl has had vomiting and diarrhoea for 1 day. She is drowsy and does not respond to voice, but flexes and moans when a cannula is inserted. She is moderately dehydrated. She has a capillary blood glucose of 1.6mmol/L and no ketones in her urine.

33. A 4-year-old girl with type 1 diabetes is in diabetic ketoacidosis. She is treated for cardiovascular shock and started on an insulin infusion. Six hours later, she becomes unresponsive, bradycardic, and hypertensive.

34. A 4-year-old boy with sickle cell disease has fluctuating consciousness. He has a headache and weakness of his right arm and leg.

35. A term baby is born by emergency caesarian section after failure to progress in labour. The cardiotocograph (CTG) showed decreased variability and late decelerations for 2h prior to delivery. At birth, he is floppy, intermittently arches and extends his body, and does not suck.

Causes of discoloured urine

For each child presenting with red urine, choose the *single* most likely diagnosis from the list of options below. Each option may be used once, more than once, or not at all. ★ ★

A Alport's syndrome

B Coagulopathy

C Drug side effect

D Fictitious

E Haemoglobinuria

F Henoch–Schönlein purpura

G Post-infectious glomerulonephritis

H Stones in urinary tract

I Thin basement membrane

J Trauma

K Tumour in urinary tract

L Urate crystals

M Urinary tract infection

36. A 4-month-old baby has had some orange-red stains in his wet nappy over the past 24h. His parents have never noticed this before. He has had a runny nose for the past 3 weeks, but is otherwise well and thriving. He is breastfed. Examination is normal. Urine dipstick is negative for glucose, blood, protein, ketones, leucocytes, and nitrites.

37. A 4-year-old boy has had dark urine for 3 days. He is otherwise well. He was unwell 2 weeks ago with a cough, cold, and sore throat, and had a course of amoxicillin. Examination is normal, except for several mobile, upper cervical lymph nodes. His blood pressure is 110/53mmHg. A urine dipstick shows 2+ blood and 1+ protein.

38. A 10-month-old baby has a fever of 39°C and is irritable. He has had two previous episodes of fever when there was no obvious cause, but no tests were done. He appears miserable and has several mobile, upper cervical lymph nodes. A urine dipstick shows 2+ blood, 1+ protein, 3+ leucocytes, and 2+ nitrites.

39. A 5-year-old girl has had red urine for 24h. Both her parents have had colds recently and her 2-year-old brother was admitted to hospital 2 days ago with suspected meningitis, for which the whole family have been given an antibiotic. A urine dipstick is negative.

40. A 10-year-old boy has been followed up in paediatric outpatients because dipsticks of his urine have been persistently positive for blood (usually 1+), but otherwise negative. The first dipstick was done 1 year ago when he had enuresis. Urine culture was negative and microscopy showed red cells but no casts. All further blood tests and a renal ultrasound have been normal. His enuresis has now resolved and he is otherwise well. He has never had any visible abnormality of the urine. His blood pressure is 110/62mmHg. Two family members have had longstanding isolated haematuria. There is no family history of deafness.

Causes of fits, faints, and funny turns

For each child presenting with a paroxysmal episode, choose the *single* most likely diagnosis from the list of options below. Each option may be used once, more than once, or not at all. ★ ★ ★

A Benign childhood epilepsy with centrotemporal spikes (Rolandic)

B Breath-holding attack

C Childhood absence epilepsy

D Juvenile myoclonic epilepsy

E Night terrors

F Pseudo-seizure

G Self-gratification phenomenon

H Syncope

I Temporal lobe epilepsy

J West syndrome (infantile spasms)

41. A 10-month-old boy is having episodes where he suddenly jerks his head forwards and extends his arms upwards. He was sitting on his own 2 months ago, but now needs support to sit. His babbling has reduced. His electroencephalogram (EEG) has a chaotic appearance.

42. A 15-month-old girl has had ten episodes over the past 2 months when she suddenly becomes silent, usually after a cry, and then becomes unconscious for a few seconds. On two occasions, there were brief clonic limb movements towards the end of the episode. She rapidly returns to normal. All of the episodes were triggered by frustration or pain. She has always been afebrile.

43. A 3-year-old girl has recurrent episodes at nursery lasting 5–10min during story time, when she becomes red and sweaty and her eyes glaze over. She is usually sitting on the mat with her legs outstretched and her body rocks backwards and forwards. When picked up, she immediately returns to normal.

44. A 9-year-old boy has had three episodes that occur on waking. He first feels a tingling on one side of the mouth and then makes a gurgling noise and cannot speak properly. He then gets small jerking movements, which spread from his arm to his leg on the left side. Afterwards, he is sleepy for a few hours.

45. A 12-year-old girl 'goes blank' for several seconds at a time 20 or 30 times in the school day. Afterwards, she has lost the thread of any conversation or class discussion. She tends to have small, repetitive hand movements during these episodes.

ANSWERS

Single Best Answers

1. E ★   OHCS 8th edn → p136

Heart murmurs are heard in many neonates. It is important to know the characteristics that signify congenital heart disease. Significant murmurs are usually harsh sounding and may be associated with thrills. In this case, the systolic murmur indicates a lesion where turbulent flow occurs in systole, i.e. aortic stenosis, pulmonary stenosis, ventricular septal defect, and atrial septal defect. The thrill at the left sternal edge indicates turbulent flow in the area of the septum. A patent ductus has a continuous murmur as blood flows across the ductus in both systole and diastole. Normal femoral pulses point against a severe aortic stenosis or coarctation.

2. E ★   OHCS 8th edn → p151

The mild upper respiratory symptoms are not a reason to delay. The red area and irritability after the previous immunization is normal, and she should have been counselled to expect this.

→ http://www.dh.gov.uk/en/Publichealth/Healthprotection/ Immunisation/Greenbook/index.htm? ('The Green Book'; see Chapter 6. This is a key UK resource for immunization.)

3. E ★   OHCS 8th edn → pp188–189

This child has diabetic ketoacidosis. Fluid management has been appropriate so far, but now that she has passed urine, she needs potassium adding to her maintenance fluid, otherwise she will quickly become hypokalaemic. Her glucose is falling at a rate of 2.5mmol/h, which is about right. You do not want it to fall faster than 5mmol/h. Once her blood glucose reaches 14–17mmol/L, you would change her IV fluid to one containing dextrose and potassium. The slight fall in her calcium is not significant.

4. C ★

A common mistake in management of constipation is to discontinue the laxative too quickly. It should have been continued for about 6 months to allow time for the distended 'baggy' colon to return to normal, and this needs to be explained to the parents at the outset. This girl's constipation has relapsed, and her soiling is due to overflow. Suppositories should be avoided in young children if at all possible. Movicol® is an osmotic laxative (containing ethylene glycol particles).
→ http://adc.bmj.com/cgi/content/full/94/2/156

5. B ★   OHCS 8th edn → p211

This is primary mono-symptomatic nocturnal enuresis, and he should do well with an enuresis alarm. He should be followed up every few weeks while using it. He has not made progress over 4 weeks with a star chart, so it is best not to persist with this on its own, but it could be combined with alarm treatment. Desmopressin could be used in the short term if he is not dry by the time of the cub camp. Imipramine is a second-line drug treatment because of the higher incidence of side effects. Oxybutynin would only be appropriate if there were symptoms of detrusor instability (e.g. daytime urgency and frequency). Enuresis is common and the National Institute for Health and Clinical Excellence (NICE) are releasing guidelines for England and Wales in 2010.

6. C ★   OHCS 8th edn → p234

This child is moderately dehydrated due to gastroenteritis, and should have an initial trial of oral rehydration therapy (ORT), especially as he is not vomiting. Aim for him to drink 20mL/kg/h. If he is not managing to drink this, then change to nasogastric ORT. If he is vomiting, then use IV fluid. If he was severely dehydrated, you would initially give 20ml/kg IV 0.9% saline.
→ http://www.bmj.com/cgi/content/full/334/7583/35?grp = 1

7. B ★

Up to 60% of newborn infants have audible but benign heart murmurs in the first 24h of life. They are due to the increase in pulmonary blood flow that occurs after birth in association with relatively high pulmonary vascular resistance. As the pulmonary vascular resistance drops, the murmur disappears.

8. D ★ OHCS 8th edn → p166

This child has signs of a flitting polyarthritis – arthritis affecting more than four joints that comes and goes. She also has the rash of erythema marginatum. Coupled with the recent history of a sore throat, this fits the criteria for rheumatic fever. You need two major criteria (of which both of these fit) or one major and two minor criteria (fever is a minor criterion). Rheumatic fever is less common now in the UK, possibly due to the use of antibiotics for streptococcal throat infections. However, it is still seen in other parts of the world. It is caused by a cross-sensitivity reaction to Group A *Streptococcus* in susceptible people.

9. A ★ OHCS 8th edn → p170

Appendicitis is the commonest cause of acute abdomen and should not be forgotten in children. It is rare under 5 years and gets more common as the child gets older. The classical presentation is central, colicky abdominal pain, which then spreads to the right iliac fossa and becomes constant in nature. However, the pain may not always be in a classical position, so other clues need to be looked for. Vomiting is almost universal, plus associated anorexia. Loose stool and dysuria may occur because of irritation from the inflamed appendix, so in a child with other symptoms do not automatically presume a simple gastroenteritis or urinary tract infection.

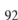

10. B ★ OHCS 8th edn → p684

Barlow's and Ortolani's tests are the way to check for developmental dysplasia of the hip. Barlow's should be done first. Barlow's = Back; hold the thigh in one hand whilst stabilizing the pelvis with the other; with the leg in the midline, push back gently. If the hip is dislocatABLE, the femoral head will pop out of the acetabulum. Ortolani's test = Out; holding the leg in the same way, gently and steadily abduct the leg as far as you can, pushing up gently with your fingers on the greater trochanter. If the hip is dislocatED you will feel the femoral head pop back into the acetabulum, or the hip will simply not abduct fully.

11. D ★ OHCS 8th edn → pp220–221

→ http://www.gpnotebook.co.uk/simplepage.cfm?ID=1946550277

12. C ★

As the law stands, children under the age of 16 can consent to treatment if judged to be Gillick competent, but cannot refuse treatment. A person with parental responsibility consents on behalf of children under 16. As the mother is the only person with parental responsibility, she is the person who should decide future treatment.

However, in practice, all effort is made to help all parties reach a decision together.

→ http://www.gmc-uk.org/guidance/ethical_guidance/children_guidance/index.asp

13. A ★   OHCS 8th edn → p136

This describes heart failure: shortness of breath and sweating, worse on effort such as feeding, tachypnoea, tachycardia, and hepatomegaly. He is also showing signs of shock. Heart failure often presents in neonates at about 4–6 weeks of age when the pulmonary vascular resistance falls.

14. B ★

Babies are allowed to lose up to 10% of their birth weight in the first week and should have regained their birth weight by 2 weeks of age. This baby has lost 150g, which is 5.5% of 2.7kg. Although breastfeeding was slow at the start in this baby, it is now going well and should be encouraged.

15. A ★   OHCS 8th edn → p166

Children who have congenital heart lesions are at risk of infective endocarditis. Poor dental hygiene is a risk factor.

16. D ★

The features point to a diagnosis of rickets. This is especially common in African-Caribbean and South Asian children in the UK who are breastfed for a prolonged period. This is because dark-skinned people absorb less sunlight and there is less conversion of 7-dehydrocholesterol to pre-vitamin D_3. This results in even lower levels of vitamin D in breast milk.

17. C ★   OHCS 8th edn → p146

The concern here is of non-accidental injury. In thinking about the mechanism of an injury, it is vital always to consider the child's developmental stage – can a 7-month-old child climb out of a cot?

18. E ★   OHCS 8th edn → p162

It is important always to reconsider a diagnosis of 'asthma' in children who do not respond to treatment and to consider referral for specialist opinion. In this case, the recurrent infections, nasal discharge, poor growth, and clubbing suggest cystic fibrosis. A sweat test is diagnostic for this and should be done. Lung function and a CT scan of the chest may be performed following diagnosis for added information, but the important step is making the diagnosis.

→ http://www.library.nhs.uk/geneticconditions/ViewResource.aspx?resID=83901

19. B ★   OHCS 8th edn → pp178–179

Nephrotic syndrome is a triad of hypoalbuminaemia, proteinuria, and oedema. It often presents with periorbital oedema just after a viral infection and it is important to dip a urine sample to look for the proteinuria or it may be dismissed as an allergic reaction, of which angioedema may be a variety. The lack of blood in the urine rules out glomerulonephritis, and SLE is rare. The presence of oedema rules out benign postural proteinuria.

20. E ★

Tension pneumothorax must always be considered in acutely ill asthmatic patients who deteriorate suddenly.

21. B ★   OHCS 8th edn → pp188–189

In any sick child remember ABCDEFG: Airway, Breathing, Circulation and Don't Ever Forget Glucose. This girl is shocked, dehydrated, and has altered consciousness and a relative hyponatraemia and hyperkalaemia caused by hyperglycaemia. The diagnosis is diabetic ketoacidosis, and a capillary blood glucose test will confirm this.

22. A ★   OHCS 8th edn → p158

This child is very likely to have epiglottitis; he has not been immunized so is not protected against *Haemophilus influenzae* type B and he has signs of upper airway obstruction. Any disturbance may cause deterioration, and an attempt to examine the throat may cause fatal respiratory arrest. Intubation is made difficult due to the swollen epiglottis, and occasionally emergency tracheostomy is required. Senior anaesthetic and ENT help should be summoned urgently.

23. D ★   OHCS 8th edn → p206; OHP → p506

There seems to be developmental regression (at least for gross motor), which would not be consistent with a febrile convulsion. Other more serious diagnoses should be considered.

24. D ★   OHCS 8th edn → p596

This is a severe case of seborrhoeic dermatitis affecting the scalp (also known as 'cradle cap' in young children). Note the thick yellow scale and crust.

25. B ★ ★

The benefits of breast milk by far outweigh the disadvantages of mild jaundice. Although it is not totally clear why breastfed babies get persistent jaundice, these babies rarely, if ever, get levels of unconjugated bilirubin high enough to cause kernicterus.

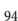

26. D ★★   OHCS 8th edn → p655

The clinical features point to Turner's syndrome: female, short stature, ptosis, and a left heart defect. This is an XO karyotype, with only one X chromosome, and is diagnosed by chromosome analysis. This should always be thought about in girls with short stature.

27. E ★★

The wrist X-ray shows widened, frayed, and cupped metaphyses of the radius and ulna. These changes are typical of rickets and are usually combined with osteopenia. The metaphysis is the growth plate and lies between the diaphysis (shaft of long bone) and epiphysis (end of the bone). This area fails to mineralize normally in the growing child due to low vitamin D levels. The aetiology is most likely to be due to a combination of initial low vitamin D stores secondary to maternal deficiency and ongoing low sunlight exposure.

28. D ★★   OHCS 8th edn → p152

These are the classic phenotypic features of a baby with trisomy 21 (Down's syndrome). The consistent neurological finding in babies with trisomy 21 is generalized hypotonia – they are floppy babies.

29. B ★★   OHCS 8th edn → p176; OHP → p384

This is haemolytic uraemic syndrome, which is usually caused by the verocytotoxin-producing *E. coli*. The toxin causes haemolysis and renal failure.

30. C ★★   OHCS 8th edn → p201

The headache is typical of migraine. The long history and lack of any suggestive features effectively rules out a space-occupying lesion. For this reason, and because there is a clear clinical diagnosis, a CT scan is not indicated. The frequency of bad attacks (more than once a month) interfering with school justifies prophylactic treatment, and pizotifen is probably most commonly used in the UK and licensed at this age. However, it is not of proven benefit. He is a too young for sumatriptan nasal spray (although this can be given orally).

→ http://ihs-classification.org/en/02_klassifikation/02_teil1/01.00.00_migraine.html (International Headache Society)

Barnes N P and Jayawant S (2005) Migraine. *Arch Dis Child Ed Pract* **90**:ep53–ep57; Ryan S (2007) Medicines for migraine. *Arch Dis Child Ed Pract* **92**:ep50–ep55.

31. E ★★   OHCS 8th edn → p180

He is most likely to have constitutional delay in growth and puberty. As testicular enlargement is the first sign of puberty in boys, measurement of testicular volume (using an orchidometer– a string of testicle-shaped beads of different volumes) will tell you if he has started puberty even in the absence of other signs. If his testicular size is greater than 4mL, then you can reassure him that he has entered puberty, and the other signs and a growth spurt will follow. The pubertal growth spurt is a late event in boys. All of the other items are relevant and should be recorded.

32. D ★★★   OHCS 8th edn → p107

Pre-term babies lose heat very easily; placing them immediately into a plastic bag has been shown to be most effective in conserving heat. Hypothermia is associated with a worse outcome and should be avoided.

33. A ★★★

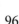

Analgesia should not be forgotten in children in pain. There is well-published guidance on a step-wise approach to analgesia, starting with simple treatments and adding in further treatment. However, different analgesics are good for different types of pain. Bony pain responds well to non-steroidal anti-inflammatory drugs (NSAIDs) and she is already on one of those so another is not appropriate. In malignancy, opioids are often needed and simple ones such as codeine should be tried first. Diazepam and hyoscine may be adjunctive treatments in symptom control in palliative care but are not analgesics. → http://www.who.int/cancer/palliative/painladder/en/index.html

34. A ★★★   OHCS 8th edn → p132

This shows epispadias, where the urethral meatus comes out on the dorsum of the penis. More common is hypospadias, where the urethral meatus comes out on the ventral aspect of the penis and is often narrowed. In reconstruction of both, the foreskin may be needed, so it is vital to warn parents not to circumcise until the surgeon has made an operative assessment. Otherwise, there is no increased risk of infection and it is always better not to retract the foreskin of babies.

35. C ★★★

Drug errors are one of the commonest type of error in paediatric practice. Everyone can make an error, and the best way to improve patient safety is to improve systems and training. Parents should receive an early explanation and apology. Any such incident is serious and you should promptly involve a senior colleague. You may think no harm has been done, but there may be wider issues to consider. Reflective portfolio entries and notifying your defence society are often appropriate but are not the most important actions.

→ http://www.npsa.nhs.uk/nrls/improvingpatientsafety/patient-safety-tools-and-guidance/beingopen/

36. B ★ ★ ★   OHCS 8th edn → p174

Note that investigation of UTIs in children has changed in England and Wales recently with the publication of the National Institute for Health and Clinical Excellence (NICE) guidelines. Investigation is generally more conservative. This child is under 6 months, but her UTI was typical and not recurrent, and she responded to treatment within 48h. Therefore, she needs a renal ultrasound, which should be performed within 6 weeks, to look for anatomical abnormalities, but does not need any other imaging.

→ http://www.nice.org.uk/Guidance/CG54

37. E ★ ★ ★   OHCS 8th edn → pp156, 186

The incidence of type 2 diabetes is rising in children, although it is still far less common than type 1 diabetes. Risk is increased in children who are overweight, have a family history of type 2 diabetes, and are of South Asian origin. The velvety skin in her axillae is acanthosis nigricans, a finding in insulin resistance and obesity.

38. E ★ ★ ★   OHCS 8th edn → p118

Surfactant treatment via an endotracheal tube is the most important treatment for respiratory distress syndrome and should be given as rescue treatment as soon as the baby has been intubated. Antibiotics should also be commenced (if not already) after blood cultures have been taken, and morphine may be needed for sedation on the ventilator.

39. A ★ ★ ★   OHCS 8th edn → p212

ADHD is part of a spectrum of hyperactive behaviour. It is characterized by lack of concentration and impulsivity, with or without hyperactivity, that is pervasive throughout all areas of the child's life. It is more common in children with learning difficulties. Autism is also part of a spectrum, characterized by impaired social interaction, impaired imagination, and a limited repertoire of interests. Dyspraxia is a developmental co-ordination disorder. Oppositional defiant disorder is a pattern of defiant, disobedient, and hostile behaviour.

40. C ★ ★ ★ ★   OHCS 8th edn → p130

This is a typical story of oesophageal atresia, with polyhydramnios, blowing bubbles, respiratory distress, and inability to pass a nasogastric tube. Approximately 92% of oesophageal atresias are also associated with a tracheo-oesophageal fistula. The H-type, where both oesophagus and trachea are patent but there is a small connection between them, is rare and is often diagnosed later.

41. E ★ ★ ★ ★ OHCS 8th edn → p601

The combination of a sick child, an erythematous rash with exfoliation, and severe mucous membrane involvement indicates Stevens–Johnson syndrome. This is associated with some viral infections and certain drugs, including penicillins.

42. E ★ ★ ★ ★ OHCS 8th edn → p638; OHP → p919

The MRI scan shows subependymal nodules in the left ventricle. This, combined with seizures and hypopigmented skin lesions, is strongly suggestive of tuberous sclerosis.

43. A ★ ★ ★ ★ OHP → p406

Catch up growth for weight in early childhood is a risk factor for obesity.
→ http://www.pubmedcentral.nih.gov/articlerender.fcgi?tool=pubme d&pubmedid=1645067

44. D ★ ★ ★ ★ OHCS 8th edn → p136

Prostaglandin E$_2$ should be commenced because the clinical presentation fits with a duct-dependent congenital cardiac lesion where the duct has just closed. This means blood can no longer flow around the body. It should cause the duct to re-open until something definitive can be done. The duct typically closes at around 48h of age, so babies who collapse at this age should always have a duct-dependent lesion considered.

45. B ★ ★ ★ ★ OHCS 8th edn → p178–179; OHP → p388

He almost certainly has minimal change nephrotic syndrome (MCNS), given his age, normal blood pressure, lack of haematuria, and normal renal function and other blood tests. For children with MCNS, 95% will respond to steroids, although most relapse at some point. The long-term outlook is good.

Eddy AA and Symons JM (2003) Nephrotic syndrome in childhood. *Lancet* **362**:629–639.

Extended Matching Questions

1. L ★

These are bright red and irregular. They enlarge in size initially and then shrink and disappear by the age of 4–5 years. They are distinguished from port-wine stains (capillary vascular naevus) as these are flat and a purplish colour, like port wine. Stork mark is the name for a capillary dilatation on the nape of the neck.

2. E ★

These are seen in over half of newborns and are caused by entrapment of fluid during development of the palate. They disappear in a few weeks and are harmless.

3. F ★

This is seen in about half of newborns and, despite the name, is totally harmless. Classically, there are small pustule-like spots on a red base and the fleeting nature is characteristic. The main differential is a staphylococcal skin infection, which has smaller, non-mobile spots.

4. K ★

5. H ★

This mark is common in dark-skinned babies and is sometimes mistaken for bruising. The blue colour is caused by melanocytes in the skin and it is usually over the lumbo-sacral area, although it can occur elsewhere.

6. E ★

The characteristic distribution of the rash on the buttocks combined with swollen joints suggests Henoch–Schönlein pupura.

7. C ★

The chronic history, loose stools, and weight loss coupled with raised inflammatory markers suggest Crohn's disease.

8. F ★

This is a surgical emergency and should be suspected in children aged 5–18 months, although it can occur at an older age. The intermittent painful episodes with pallor are classic, as is the 'redcurrant jelly' stool, although this is a late sign.

9. J ★

The long history with normal growth is very reassuring and suggests a non-organic cause.

10. A ★

This causes poor growth with malabsorption stools that are loose and bulky. Classically, it causes abdominal distension and the child is miserable. It occurs after the introduction of gluten-containing foods, but can otherwise occur at any age.

General feedback on 5–10: OHCS 8th edn → p170–172

11. D ★

Croup, or viral laryngotracheobronchitis, is common. It causes symptoms of a cold plus laryngeal oedema. This causes a harsh cough, typically barking like a seal and easy to recognize, and stridor.

12. I ★

Whooping cough has not disappeared completely, despite immunization. It occurs in young children who have not yet been fully immunized, and can be serious. The bouts of coughing are paroxysmal, severe, and prolonged, and may end in apnoea. The characteristic finding is a marked lymphocytosis on blood tests.

13. G ★

Although asthma is common, many children who are diagnosed actually have other conditions. The normal investigations and lack of family history call the diagnosis into question. The bad breath and symptoms limited to night time when lying down are clues for reflux.

14. J ★

The mucus indicates that this baby cannot swallow secretions. The choking on first feed also indicates that she is having problems swallowing. The term tracheo-oesophageal fistula refers to a number of different patterns, but the commonest types have oesophageal atresia, causing inability to swallow. In this case, there will be polyhydramnios in pregnancy because the fetus cannot swallow amniotic fluid.

15. F ★

Young children frequently inhale small objects during play, such as peanuts or small bits of toys. If this is witnessed, it is reasonably easy to make a diagnosis. Unilateral wheeze confirms the diagnosis as there is selective obstruction of the airways on one side.

General feedback on 11–15: OHCS 8th edn → pp158–160, 164

16. L ★

Prolonged rupture of membranes is a risk factor for sepsis. Poor feeding and jaundice may be signs of sepsis and this should always be considered in unwell newborns.

17. C ★

Babies with Down's syndrome are always floppy. Dysmorphic features may be subtle, such as the white flecks on the iris (Brushfield spots). Heart defects are also common in Down's syndrome.

18. E ★

This baby has Beckwith–Wiedemann syndrome, a rare overgrowth syndrome. Babies with this are large for dates, have large organs, and may have exomphalos because of bowel overgrowth. A characteristic feature is earlobe creases. They become hypoglycaemic because of increased insulin, in the same way that babies of diabetic mothers do.

19. G ★

This describes the brain damage that occurs because of oxygen deprivation at birth. This is a risk in abruption, and the poor Apgar scores indicate that this baby suffered from the start.

20. H ★

Consanguinity (having a child with a close relative) increases the risk of inborn errors of metabolism, which tend to be autosomal recessive in inheritance. They often cause hypoglycaemia and acidosis.

21. I ★

Sepsis is the main diagnosis to consider in unwell babies. Hypothermia can be seen rather than fever, and a range of metabolic disturbances. This baby is shocked and unwell.

22. F ★

Bloody diarrhoea, weight loss, and anaemia all indicate a significant pathology. There are signs of inflammation on blood tests with elevated white cell count and platelets.

23. B ★

The timing of change in milk is important here.

24. A ★

Type 1 diabetes is an autoimmune condition and there is increased risk of other immune-mediated diseases such as coeliac disease, which is characterized by features of malabsorption.

25. J ★

Following gastroenteritis, the gut can take time to heal and there may be a transient lactose intolerance. This will cause symptoms of malabsorption.

General feedback on 21–25: OHCS 8th edn → pp168, 171

26. F ★

Duchenne's muscular dystrophy affects boys and usually presents at around 1–6 years with weakness and waddling gait. These boys often have motor developmental delay and may walk late.

27. A ★

Premature babies are at increased risk of spastic diplegia, a form of cerebral palsy affecting the lower limbs more than the upper limbs. There is delayed development and hypertonia, causing scissoring of the legs.

28. H ★

This is an osteochondritis of the femoral head and is seen mainly in 4–7 year olds, and in boys more than girls. It causes a painful limp with limited hip movement. The normal blood tests rule out leukaemia or idiopathic thrombocytopaenic purpura. Slipped upper femoral epiphysis is painless and occurs in older children.

29. J ★

This is rare and causes neurological and liver abnormalities, which may not be seen at the same time. It occurs in older children.

30. C ★

The classical presentation of Henoch–Schönlein purpura is a purpuric rash on the lower limbs and buttocks of a well child, who also has joint pain and swelling. It typically occurs a few weeks after a viral illness, although the cause is unknown.

General feedback on 26–30: OHCS 8th edn → pp214, 642, 682

31. B ★

The rash looks viral in nature here and is likely to be caused by herpes simplex virus, which can cause encephalitis.

32. C ★

Inborn errors of metabolism can present in many ways but should be considered in infants who present with decreased consciousness. The clues here are hypoglycaemia without ketones, meaning that the body needs fuel but cannot mount the normal metabolic pathways and produce ketones.

33. A ⋆

Cerebral oedema is a recognized risk in diabetic ketoacidosis if too much fluid is given too rapidly. It is important to treat shock, but fluid management needs to be meticulous.

34. I ⋆

Sickle cell disease causes blockage of the small blood vessels as the sickled cells cannot flow smoothly. In the brain, this can lead to areas of ischaemia and stroke.

35. D ⋆

An abnormal CTG is an indication of hypoxia *in utero*.

General feedback on 31–35: OHCS 8th edn → pp183, 189, 202

36. L ⋆⋆

Urate crystals can sometimes look like blood stains on the nappy, but usually have an orange-red quality that is quite characteristic. If there is any doubt, the red area can be eluted into some water in a specimen pot and tested with a urine dipstick, which will indicate the presence of any blood. The test will be negative if urate crystals are the cause.

37. G ⋆⋆

This is typical of post-streptococcal glomerulonephritis. Note that the antistreptolysin O titre is raised. The urine is typically described as 'smoky' or like 'Coca Cola'.

38. M ⋆⋆

The urine dipstick strongly suggests a urinary tract infection (UTI). The two previous febrile episodes may also have been UTIs. Consider looking for other causes of fever in a young child who is irritable with a high fever, including septicaemia and meningitis (depending on how ill the child appears).

39. C ⋆⋆

This child is being treated with rifampicin as meningococcal prophylaxis. This drug can turn the urine pink, and the parents should have been warned about this.

40. I ⋆⋆

Isolated persistent haematuria with minimal or no proteinuria, normal renal function, and with a family history of similar benign problems suggests thin basement membrane disease, otherwise known as benign familial haematuria. Make sure there is no family history of deafness (which suggests Alport's syndrome) or renal failure (which might indicate a more serious cause).

General feedback on 36–40: OHCS 8th edn → pp174, 178

41. J ★ ★ ★

West syndrome is otherwise known as infantile spasms, so the age is a pointer. The flexor spasms, developmental regression, and characteristic electroencephalogram (EEG) appearance (hypsarrhythmia) all point to the diagnosis.

42. B ★ ★ ★

The fact that all episodes are triggered by frustration or pain makes epilepsy very unlikely and points strongly to breath-holding. The age and description is typical. Brief clonic movements may occur.

43. G ★ ★ ★

This is a form of masturbation. The age and description are typical, as is the fact that she returns to normal when self-stimulation is prevented.

44. A ★ ★ ★

Nocturnal seizures that progress from arm to leg on one side are typical of this condition.

45. C ★ ★ ★

Absences are described, and the small movements (which can also be around the face or lips) are a helpful clue (although not always present).

General feedback on 40–45: OHCS 8th edn → pp206–207

CHAPTER 3

PSYCHIATRY

Dinesh Bhugra, Gill McGauley, and Isobel McMullen

Mental health problems are estimated to affect one in four people each year in the UK, making mental illness one of the most common presentations to GP surgeries, outpatient clinics, and Emergency Departments. Yet many doctors and medical students feel uncertain about how to approach patients with psychiatric disorder.

The key to becoming a good psychiatrist is in the clinical interview. There are few physical signs or investigations that allow doctors to diagnose psychiatric illness, so a detailed history and mental state examination is important. As a psychiatrist, you are in the privileged position of having patients tell you their personal stories, and the skill is in listening attentively and asking relevant questions to help clarify parts of the story. The best way to practise these techniques is to watch experienced clinicians at work and interview patients yourself.

Obviously diagnosis is important, so you need to be aware of the types of symptoms that fit with each type of disorder, as well as medical conditions that may mimic psychiatric illness. Investigations may be necessary to rule out other diseases and you need to be able to request these appropriately. Psychiatrists have access to a range of treatments, and you need to know which to recommend: medical (such as antidepressants), psychological (such as cognitive behavioural therapy), and physical (such as electroconvulsive therapy). Most of these are delivered in conjunction with the multidisciplinary team, so you should be clear about the roles of each team member.

Finally, there is overlap between psychiatry and the law, which can raise interesting ethical issues. Treating someone against their will is sometimes necessary for their safety or the safety of others, so you need to know about mental health law. Psychiatrists are also often requested to provide a second opinion about difficult capacity decisions. ■

Isobel McMullen

PSYCHIATRY
SINGLE BEST ANSWERS

1. A 53-year-old builder has injured his arm and is admitted to the ward. Late one night, he becomes aggressive, shouting at the nurses and other patients, wanting to leave the ward, and saying that he can see ants running all over the walls. Which is the single most likely cause of these symptoms? ★

A Abnormal reaction to analgesic medication

B Alcohol withdrawal

C Dissocial personality disorder

D Head injury

E Past history of schizophrenia

2. A 20-year-old woman took 40 paracetamol tablets 9h ago. Which is the single most appropriate emergency treatment? ★

A Activated charcoal

B Diazepam

C Flumazenil

D *N*-Acetylcysteine

E Naloxone

3. A 34-year-old woman has severe abdominal pain and blood in her stool. Abdominal and pelvic examinations are normal, except for multiple surgical scars over the abdomen consistent with laparoscopies and an appendicectomy. She gives stool samples from home with blood in but has not managed to produce one in hospital. Blood and urine investigations are normal, but she insists on further investigation and does not want to leave hospital. Which is the single most likely diagnosis? ★

A Delusional disorder

B Hypochondriacal disorder

C Malingering

D Mild–moderate depressive episode

E Munchausen syndrome

4. A 25-year-old man is disorientated and has slurred speech and respiratory depression. He has miosis. Which is the single most likely cause? ★

A Alcohol abuse

B Carbon monoxide poisoning

C Opioid abuse

D Paracetamol overdose

E Salicylate overdose

5. A 36-year-old man goes to a plastic surgeon insisting on surgery, saying that his nose is too big and crooked. He says that people stare at him when he goes out, so he prefers not to leave the house. He feels depressed as a result. He attributes his recent job loss to his 'deformed nose'. He wears make-up to camouflage it, but would like surgery to correct what appears to be a normal nose. Which is the single most likely diagnosis? ★

A Body dysmorphic disorder

B Hypochondriasis

C Mild–moderate depressive episode

D Obsessive–compulsive disorder

E Social phobia

6. A 61-year-old man attends his GP at the request of his wife who thinks he drinks too much alcohol. Which single factor is a sign of alcohol dependence? ★

A A wide repertoire of alcoholic drinks

B Decreased tolerance to alcohol

C Drinking 28 units of alcohol or more a week

D Drinking despite evidence of its harm to job and family

E Drinking until late in the evening

7. A 20-year-old man has a first episode of psychosis. Your consultant asks you to prescribe an atypical (or second-generation) antipsychotic. Which single drug should be prescribed? ★

A Chlorpromazine

B Haloperidol

C Lorazepam

D Mirtazapine

E Olanzapine

8. A 64-year-old man is recovering after a myocardial infarction (MI). His recovery is slowed by poor sleep, loss of appetite, lack of motivation, and feelings of hopelessness. Your consultant believes he is depressed and asks you to commence antidepressant treatment. He has no other medical history. Which would be the single most appropriate class of drug to prescribe? ★

A Benzodiazepine

B Monoamine oxidase inhibitor (MAOI)

C Selective serotonin reuptake inhibitor (SSRI)

D Serotonin and noradrenaline (norepinephrine) reuptake inhibitor

E Tricyclic antidepressant

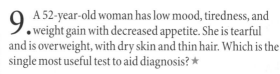

9. A 52-year-old woman has low mood, tiredness, and weight gain with decreased appetite. She is tearful and is overweight, with dry skin and thin hair. Which is the single most useful test to aid diagnosis? ★

A Chest X-ray

B Electrocardiogram

C Full blood count

D Thyroid function tests

E Urea and electrolytes

10. A 35-year-old woman suddenly starts to feel dizzy and short of breath, with chest pains and a tingling sensation in her fingers. Symptoms worsen until she feels as if she is about to die. It lasts about 10 min before resolving completely. Which is the single most likely diagnosis? ★

A Acute asthma

B Myocardial infarction

C Panic attack

D Temporal lobe epilepsy

E Transient ischaemic attack

11. A 36-year-old woman is 36 weeks pregnant with twins. She has obsessive–compulsive disorder. She is scheduled to have an elective caesarean section for the delivery of her twins due to complications in her last delivery and pre-eclampsia in this pregnancy. She has already consented to the operation. She has now become agitated and anxious and is refusing to co-operate, saying that she does not want to have the operation and wants to go home. Which is the single most appropriate course of action? ★

A Arrange emergency detention under the Mental Health Act 2007 (England and Wales) as it is necessary for her health to be treated

B Assess her capacity to consent and discuss the situation with a senior doctor

C Detain her for treatment as she has a mental disorder as defined by the Mental Health Act 2007 (England and Wales)

D Prescribe sedative medication and advise the nurses to call when she is less agitated

E Tell the nurses to reassure her and carry on, as she has previously consented

12. A 44-year-old woman has taken an overdose of 20 paracetamol. Which single factor indicates the highest risk of her going on to complete suicide? ★

A Having a psychotic illness

B Living with a partner

C Taking alcohol with the overdose

D Taking more than 50 tablets as an overdose

E Writing a suicide note before the overdose

13. A 58-year-old woman has gastritis. Her GP is concerned about her possible heavy use of alcohol and arranges some screening questionnaires and blood tests. Which single result would indicate possible problem or hazardous drinking? ★

A A decreased mean corpuscular volume (MCV)

B A low level of gamma-glutamyltranspeptidase (GGT)

C A score of 5 on the Alcohol Use Disorders Identification Test (AUDIT)

D One positive reply on the CAGE questionnaire

E Raised urate levels

14. A 34-year-old man is brought to the Emergency Department by the police. He is agitated and elated. His blood pressure is 140/90mmHg, his pulse rate is 120bpm, and his pupils are dilated. Which single substance is he most likely to have been using? ★

A Cocaine

B Heroin

C Organic solvents

D Oxazepam

E Psilocybin

15. A 68-year-old man has a prominent impairment of recent memory with intact immediate recall. He has no evidence of generalized cognitive impairment and no impairment in his level of consciousness. Which is the single most likely diagnosis? ★

A Alzheimer's disease

B Delirium

C Korsakoff's syndrome

D Normal pressure hydrocephalus

E Post-ictal state

16. A 74-year-old woman has bowel cancer. The surgeons say she requires surgery, which is potentially curative, and without it she will die. The woman is refusing any surgical intervention. She had post-natal depression 42 years ago but is not currently suffering from any mental illness. Her current mini mental state score is 29/30. She knows about her diagnosis, believes it applies to her, understands the risks and benefits of the proposed surgery, and is able to retain the information. Which is the single most appropriate course of action? ★

A Detain her under a section of the Mental Health Act 2007 (England and Wales) and perform the operation

B Discharge her from hospital

C Gain a second opinion, and if they feel she has capacity, comply with her wishes

D Restrain her under common law and perform the operation

E Use the Mental Capacity Act 2005 (England and Wales) to perform the operation

17. A 40-year-old woman is having intrusive and persistent thoughts that she is a 'dirty prostitute'. She recognizes her thoughts as silly but still feels ashamed of them. Although these thoughts get her down, she still enjoys life. Which is the single most likely diagnosis? ★

A Depressive disorder

B Generalized anxiety disorder

C Obsessive–compulsive disorder

D Psychotic episode

E Schizophrenia

18. A 28-year-old man is found in an alleyway in a semi-conscious state. He has a respiratory rate of 6/min, a pulse rate of 50bpm, and pin-point pupils. Which is the single most appropriate drug to give? ★

A Clonidine

B Methadone

C Naloxone

D Naltrexone

E Thiamine

19. An 82-year-old man is forgetful, gets lost when out, and has difficulty finding his way home. On occasion, he puts his keys in the microwave and doesn't seem to know how to use it. His memory problems seemed to get markedly worse around the time he was admitted to hospital 2 years ago with a stroke, and again earlier this year when he couldn't talk for a few minutes. His speech has since recovered. Which is the single most likely diagnosis? ★

A Alzheimer's disease

B Fronto-temporal dementia

C Lewy body dementia

D Normal ageing

E Vascular dementia

20. A 28-year-old woman has low mood and loss of appetite. She is still coping at work, but lacks energy and feels her concentration is not as good as before. Her sleep is normal, and she enjoys spending time with her friends. She has never had any ideas of self-harm or suicide. Which is the single most appropriate course of action? ★

A Ask her to keep a mood diary and return to see you in 2 weeks

B Prescribe citalopram and see her again in 2 weeks

C Prescribe moclobemide and see her again in 4 weeks

D Refer her for cognitive behavioural therapy

E Tell her not to worry, and that it's normal to feel like this

21. A 29-year-old woman has recently been diagnosed as having generalized anxiety disorder. Which is the single best initial approach to management? ★

A Advise her to keep a diary of when she feels anxious

B Explain the condition to her, writing down the essential points

C Give her a standard information leaflet

D Provide information on the medication that can be used

E Recommend a self-help book

22. A 48-year-old man with alcohol dependence has been found wandering in the street. He has some clouding of consciousness, nystagmus, and opthalmoplegia. Which is the single most appropriate medication to administer initially? ★

A Acamprosate

B Disulfiram

C Metoclopramide

D Naloxone

E Thiamine

23. A 30-year-old woman with panic disorder has been treated with cognitive behavioural therapy, which has only partially helped her symptoms. She requests further treatment and is prescribed citalopram. Which is the single most likely side effect profile she should be warned about? ★

A Confusion and memory problems

B Drowsiness, palpitations, and postural hypotension

C Dry mouth, blurred vision, and constipation

D Nausea, gastrointestinal upset, restlessness, and insomnia

E Weight gain

24. A 28-year-old man who has recently been diagnosed with paranoid schizophrenia is started on risperidone. Which single common potential side effect should he be advised about? ★

A Feeling more alert

B Gynaecomastia

C Hirsutism

D Improved sexual performance

E Weight loss

25. A 67-year-old man was diagnosed with dementia a year ago. He has previously been advised, verbally and in writing, to inform the Driver and Vehicle Licensing Agency (DVLA) of his diagnosis. He says that he has not taken this advice as he needs his car to get the shops and to see his friends. On mini mental state examination, he is not disorientated but shows mild short-term memory loss. Which is the single most appropriate course of action? ★ ★

A Advise him again verbally that he needs to inform the DVLA

B Advise him verbally of your responsibility to disclose to the DVLA

C Advise him verbally that he should stop driving from now

D Disclose his diagnosis to the DVLA

E Write to him again advising that he needs to inform the DVLA

26. A 20-year-old woman has panic attacks when she has to attend formal meetings at her work. She also feels anxious when she meets her friends in the pub. Which is the single most likely diagnosis? ★ ★

A Adjustment disorder

B Generalized anxiety disorder

C Panic disorder

D Post-traumatic stress disorder

E Social phobia

27. A 60-year-old man asks for a repeat prescription of diazepam. He says that his GP started him on this treatment 3 months ago when he was anxious and depressed after losing his job. Which is the single most appropriate course of action? ★ ★

A Call his usual GP to arrange an appointment for him in a week

B Change his prescription to an antidepressant drug and explain that this would be a more appropriate treatment

C Explain that you cannot re-prescribe diazepam because of the risk of him becoming dependent

D Explain the risk of becoming dependent on diazepam and then re-prescribe diazepam at half the dose for 4 more weeks

E Explain the risk of becoming dependent on diazepam and then re-prescribe diazepam in a weekly decreasing dose

28. A 33-year-old woman with bipolar affective disorder is due to be started on a mood stabilizer. She has some questions about lithium. Which single symptom or sign is a common side effect of lithium at therapeutic levels? ★ ★

A Coarse tremor

B Dysarthria

C Improvement of pre-existing skin conditions

D Thirst

E Weight loss

29. A 24-year-old man is found acting strangely in the park. He believes that MI5 are behind a plot to harm him and are keeping him under surveillance. He hears himself being commented on by a voice 'reading the news' and thinks that his thoughts are being controlled by devices on buses. Which single symptom is one of Schneider's first-rank symptoms of schizophrenia? ★ ★

A Catatonia

B Ideas of reference

C Persecutory delusions

D Poverty of speech

E Third-person auditory hallucinations

30. A 26-year-old woman has emotional lability and a mildly depressed mood. She feels 'numb' and 'empty' and in recent times has often acted impulsively, for example by shoplifting. She uses recreational drugs regularly. She has no regular partner and is unemployed. She cuts herself in response to distressing feelings, but is not suicidal. Which is the single most likely diagnosis? ★ ★

A Antisocial personality disorder

B Avoidant personality disorder

C Emotionally unstable personality disorder

D Histrionic personality disorder

E Mild depressive episode

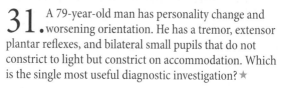

31. A 79-year-old man has personality change and worsening orientation. He has a tremor, extensor plantar reflexes, and bilateral small pupils that do not constrict to light but constrict on accommodation. Which is the single most useful diagnostic investigation? ★

A Chest X-ray

B CT scan of the brain

C Electroencephalogram

D MRI of the brain

E Venereal Disease Research Laboratory (VDRL) test

32. The police bring a 23-year-old man to the Emergency Department, who they have detained because he was standing in the middle of the road shouting at the traffic and threatening to stab drivers. The doctor is asked to take a history and examine the patient. Which is the single most appropriate initial action for the doctor to take? ★

A Arrange for the interview to take place in a quiet, private room

B Ask the police to be present during the interview

C Remove any sharp items from the room that could be used as weapons

D Talk to the police about the patient's presentation and behaviour

E Tell another member of staff to note down where the interview will take place

33. The wife of a patient is in a distressed state. She tells her GP that her husband is wandering around the house at night and she is frightened to sleep in case he accidentally harms himself. She says that her husband has already drawn up a Personal Welfare Lasting Power of Attorney (LPA), which is registered at the Office of the Public Guardian, and that he has appointed her as his 'attorney' to make decisions on his behalf. The GP knows that her husband has a diagnosis of dementia, although it is 6 months since he last saw him. The wife asks him to prescribe some sedative medication, adding that her husband is quite happy to take a tablet at night. Which is the single most appropriate response for the GP to make? ★ ★ ★

A Advise the wife that he would need to talk to other members of the family as well before he prescribed any medication

B Explain to the wife that an LPA does not cover decisions about medical treatment

C Explain to the wife that he would need to see her husband to assess whether he lacks the capacity to decide whether or not to take sedative medication

D Explain to the wife that she cannot give consent on behalf of her husband for him to prescribe medication

E Prescribe a small dose of sedative medication for the patient and see him in a week

34. A 23-year-old woman has had psychological and somatic symptoms of anxiety for 3 weeks, which mostly occur when she has to drive her car in the city. This is the first time she has suffered from these symptoms. Which is the single most appropriate treatment? ★ ★ ★ ★

A Anxiety management training

B Behavioural therapy

C Brief psychodynamic psychotherapy

D Selective serotonin reuptake inhibitor (SSRI)

E Tricyclic antidepressant

35. A 3-year-old boy has been referred to the paediatrician and child psychiatrist for assessment. He was late to talk and is falling behind his peers at nursery. He is thought to have mild learning disability. His parents have some questions. Which single statement about mild learning disability is appropriate when counselling the parents? ★ ★ ★ ★

A A specific cause cannot be identified in 50% of cases

B Epilepsy occurs in 70% of people with mild learning disability

C Fragile X syndrome is an X-linked recessive condition that can cause mild learning disability

D Only very few people are capable of working during adult life

E The expected IQ range is between 20 and 35

Psychiatry

36. A 6-year-old boy does not talk and will not play with other children. He is only interested in toy cars, and lines them up in a particular order. His teacher says he cannot read or write like the other children and has temper tantrums for no obvious reason. Which is the single most likely diagnosis? ★ ★ ★ ★

A Asperger's syndrome

B Autism

C Normal child

D Obsessive–compulsive disorder

E Rett's syndrome

37. A 30-year-old man with paranoid schizophrenia has not responded to two consecutive 8-week trials of olanzapine and risperidone at therapeutic doses. Which is the single most appropriate course of action? ★ ★ ★ ★

A Combine olanzapine and risperidone

B Commence clozapine

C Commence haloperidol

D Commence risperidone long-acting injection

E Continue olanzapine at a higher dose

38. A 35-year-old man was prescribed an antidepressant 8 months ago for a moderately severe depressive episode. This was his first depressive episode. He now feels that he has almost recovered, and wants to know when he can stop his antidepressants. Which is the single most appropriate piece of advice? ★ ★ ★ ★

A He must take the tablets for the rest of his life

B He should continue medication for 1–2 months after recovery

C He should continue medication for 4–6 months after recovery

D He should continue medication for 1 year after recovery

E He should stop the antidepressants immediately if he feels back to normal

39. A 30-year-old man with paranoid schizophrenia on the ward becomes very agitated one night. He is pacing around, talking to himself and appears to be responding to hallucinations. He is verbally aggressive and hostile to staff and other patients. He has a history of violence when unwell. Simple de-escalation techniques have failed to calm the situation down, but he is willing to take medication. Which is the single most appropriate management? ★ ★ ★ ★

A Give clozapine 50mg orally and review in 1h

B Give haloperidol 10mg IM and review in 1h

C Give lorazepam 20mg orally and review in 1h

D Give olanzapine 20mg IM and review in 1h

E Request police presence on the ward

40. A 31-year-old single mother discloses that she regularly cuts herself in front of her 6-year-old son, and that he often becomes distressed if he thinks she is feeling sad. She is not taking him to school every day. Which is the single most appropriate course of action? ★ ★ ★ ★

A Contact the school to find out if her son's teacher has any concerns about him and document the discussion

B Find out if she has any extra support, such as a family member, who could come and help out with looking after him

C Inform the police and social services immediately

D Speak to a senior colleague and the designated child protection lead at the trust

E Tell her that if she does not stop self-harming in front of him, you will have to take action

41. A 22-year-old woman has recurrent depressive episodes. Her main symptoms are low mood, anhedonia, insomnia, and weight loss secondary to poor appetite. She has had adverse reactions to selective serotonin reuptake inhibitors (SSRIs) in the past. Which would be the single most appropriate medication to prescribe? ★ ★ ★ ★

A Citalopram

B Fluoxetine

C Mirtazapine

D Paroxetine

E Sertraline

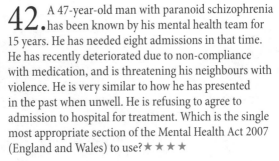

42. A 47-year-old man with paranoid schizophrenia has been known by his mental health team for 15 years. He has needed eight admissions in that time. He has recently deteriorated due to non-compliance with medication, and is threatening his neighbours with violence. He is very similar to how he has presented in the past when unwell. He is refusing to agree to admission to hospital for treatment. Which is the single most appropriate section of the Mental Health Act 2007 (England and Wales) to use? ★ ★ ★ ★

A Section 2

B Section 3

C Section 5

D Section 17

E Section 136

43. A 48-year-old woman is admitted to hospital for routine surgery. She takes once-daily lithium for treatment of bipolar disorder. Which is the single correct time to take her blood to check plasma levels of lithium? ★ ★ ★ ★

A Immediately before her dose

B 2h after her dose

C 8h after her dose

D 12h after her dose

E 20h after her dose

44. A 35-year-old man who is opiate dependent is considering tackling his addiction. In discussing treatment options, which is the single most appropriate piece of advice to include? ★ ★ ★ ★

A Methadone has a shorter half-life than heroin

B Naltrexone is an opiate agonist, which is an alternative to methadone

C Opiate withdrawal results in death if untreated

D Opiate withdrawal causes restlessness, abdominal pain, and anxiety

E Withdrawal syndrome will begin 2–3 days after the last heroin taken

$45.$ A previously healthy 78-year-old man has a severe depressive illness. He has not responded to various treatments so far and his consultant wants to prescribe a tricyclic antidepressant. Which is the single most important investigation before commencing treatment? ★ ★ ★ ★

A CT scan of the brain

B ECG

C Full blood count

D Urea and electrolytes

E Urinalysis

EXTENDED MATCHING QUESTIONS

Causes of confusional states

For each patient, choose the *single* most likely diagnosis from the list of options below. Each option may be used once, more than once, or not at all. ★

A Alcoholic hallucinosis

B Alzheimer's disease

C Delirium

D Delirium tremens

E Depressive disorder

F Depressive pseudodementia

G Dissociative fugue

H Schizophrenia

I Subdural haematoma

J Vascular (multi-infarct) dementia

K Wernicke's encephalopathy

1. A 45-year-old man has become confused and disorientated. He was seen in the Emergency Department 3 days ago and treated for a head injury he sustained in a fight after a night of heavy drinking.

2. A 78-year-old woman has become confused, scared, and agitated on the ward. Urinalysis shows the presence of protein and blood.

3. A 55-year-old man with chronic alcohol abuse is agitated. He spent yesterday in the pub but hasn't been able to buy a drink since. He is experiencing derogatory auditory hallucinations.

4. A 65-year-old man with diabetes, ischaemic heart disease, and hypertension has had memory impairment for 6 months. His wife says that he occasionally gets confused at night.

5. A 60-year-old homeless woman is brought to the Emergency Department. She smells of alcohol, is confused, and has nystagmus and a broad-based, staggering gait.

Alcohol and drug misuse

For each clinical situation, choose the *single* most likely treatment approach from the list of options below. Each option may be used once, more than once, or not at all. ★

A Acamprosate

B Buprenorphine

C Chlordiazepoxide

D Diazepam

E Disulfiram

F Fluoxetine

G Haloperidol

H Parenteral thiamine

I Olanzapine

J Oral methadone

6. A 60-year-old man who is dependent on alcohol experienced a seizure when he was previously detoxified. He wants to undergo a further detoxification.

7. A 25-year-old man has been smoking cannabis for 6 months. He has started to become suspicious of colleagues, believing they are spying on him. He believes that they can overhear his thoughts.

8. A 50-year-old man has successfully completed an alcohol detoxification programme and starts to develop cravings for alcohol. He does not want to engage in 'talking therapies'.

9. A 45-year-old man is currently dependent on alcohol and wants to undergo outpatient detoxification.

10. A 55-year-old man with alcohol dependence is acutely confused and has ophthalmoplegia.

Causes of memory loss

For each patient, choose the *single* most likely diagnosis from the list of options below. Each option may be used once, more than once, or not at all. ★

A Alzheimer's disease

B Creutzfeldt–Jakob disease

C Depressive pseudodementia

D Huntington's disease (chorea)

E Korsakoff's syndrome

F Lewy body dementia

G Mild cognitive impairment

H Parkinson's disease

I Pick's disease

J Vascular (multi-infarct) dementia

11. An 85-year-old man has an isolated memory impairment. He scores 26/30 on mini mental state examination and his activities of daily living are unimpaired.

12. A 62-year-old man is forgetful. He cannot remember how he got to the surgery, but is able to recall an address on testing of his memory. He has gynaecomastia and palmar erythema.

13. A 70-year-old woman is convinced that her neighbours are stealing her food. She has become increasingly forgetful over the last year, but blames others when she cannot find things. She wanders at night thinking it is the daytime, and finds it difficult to button up her clothes.

14. A 73-year-old woman has had memory loss for 3 months that is worse in the morning. She is distressed by her symptoms, but responds to most questions by saying 'I don't know'.

15. A 57-year-old woman has had failing memory and a tremor of her right hand for 3 years. She is finding it harder to keep up with her husband when out walking and has trouble getting up the stairs of the bus and out of chairs.

Causes of severe behavioural disturbance

For each patient with disturbed behaviour, choose the *single* most likely diagnosis from the list of options below. Each option may be used once, more than once, or not at all. ★

A Acute psychotic episode

B Delusional disorder

C Drug-induced psychosis

D Emotionally unstable personality disorder (borderline type)

E Mania with psychotic features

F Normal grief

G Psychotic depression

H Schizoaffective disorder

I Schizophrenia

J Schizotypal personality disorder

16. A 21-year-old man has been hearing voices for 2 days that he believes belong to the FBI agents who are following him. He is scared because he thinks the FBI wants him dead and so is unable to sleep. He has no psychiatric or medical history. He uses cannabis most days and 3 days ago took what his friends think was cocaine at a party.

17. A 43-year-old woman believes her husband is about to leave her because she is a useless wife and mother. She is convinced that he is having an affair and that his family are 'against her'. She now feels that her GP is part of the plot to help him divorce her. She says she has failed and deserves to be punished. Over the past few months, she has become increasingly withdrawn and neglectful of her personal hygiene. She sleeps poorly and has lost weight. She suffered with post-natal depression after the birth of her son 5 years ago.

18. A 50-year-old man has had ideas about the police wanting to harm him for 20 years. He has a vast collection of evidence that this is the case, including his post being delivered late on significant days, silent phone calls, his water supply being 'poisoned', and a sign going up that is an anagram of his name. He has never experienced any auditory or visual hallucinations.

19. A 23-year-old woman is bothered by voices. These are a combination of derogatory comments about her and remarks about the abuse she suffered as a child. The voices do not sound real but often feel like her own thoughts being echoed aloud. She finds them distressing and copes by drinking alcohol or cutting herself.

20. A 29-year-old man has been hearing voices for the last 5 years that provide a running commentary on his actions and tell him how to live his life. He has recently started to communicate with his grandmother who died 2 years ago, and believes he is carrying out her wishes. He believes that doctors are able to hear his thoughts and so dislikes them. He does not trust people who wear red as he thinks they are part of the 'Devil's Army'.

Causes of anxiety

For each patient, choose the *single* most likely diagnosis from the list of options below. Each option may be used once, more than once, or not at all. ★ ★

A Acute stress disorder

B Agoraphobia

C Dysthymia

D Generalized anxiety disorder

E Panic attack

F Panic disorder

G Paranoid personality disorder

H Post-traumatic stress disorder

I Simple phobia

J Social phobia

21. A 22-year-old woman has recurrent 20 min episodes during which she fears she is going to die because her heart races, she has chest pain and difficulty breathing, and she feels dizzy, nauseous, and shaky. They come on in a variety of situations and she spends a lot of her life fearing the next episode.

22. A 35-year-old woman has overwhelming worries about everyday things and is unable to relax. She feels on edge all the time, although she has periods when the anxiety gets worse and she feels dizzy and gets palpitations, shortness of breath, and hot flushes.

23. A 32-year-old woman becomes very anxious in a variety of situations, such as at the supermarket or on public transport. She has shortness of breath, feels sweaty, and is fearful that she may collapse in public. As a result, she rarely leaves the house alone.

24. A 42-year-old soldier is unable to relax and is irritable since returning from conflict 5 months ago. His concentration is poor and he has problems falling asleep. He has vivid memories of a car bomb in which some of his regiment died, and he now avoids driving a car if at all possible.

25. A 27-year-old man has few friends and tries to avoid contact with people because he is worried that this will end in humiliation. He does not believe that he has anything to add to gatherings and thinks that people laugh at him behind his back. When he finds himself in such situations, he becomes sweaty, blushes, and suffers from a dry mouth and trembling.

Causes of learning disability

For each patient with learning difficulties, choose the *single* most likely diagnosis from the list of options below. Each option may be used once, more than once, or not at all. ★ ★

A Angelman's syndrome

B Down's syndrome

C Fetal alcohol syndrome

D Fragile X syndrome

E Klinefelter's syndrome

F Lesch–Nyhan syndrome

G Prader–Willi syndrome

H Rett's syndrome

I Tuberous sclerosis

J Turner's syndrome

26. A 5-year-old girl had normal development until the age of 2 years, but now has epilepsy and episodes of limb spasticity. She has involuntary hand flapping and hand wringing. Her personality has changed and she is irritable and anxious at times. Her intellectual abilities have also deteriorated and she now has a severe learning disability.

27. A 3-year-old girl with fair hair and a prominent jaw has epilepsy and severe learning disability. She is unable to walk properly due to jerky limb movements. She has episodes of uncontrolled laughter and hand flapping.

28. A 39-year-old man with lifelong short stature and moderate learning disability starts to experience difficulty in daily tasks, such as cooking, that he would previously have been able to do easily. His language skills are deteriorating and he has become more withdrawn and irritable.

29. A 3-year-old girl has short stature and low weight with microcephaly, a short palpebral fissure, and a smooth philtrum. She was late to walk and talk and is falling behind her peers at playgroup.

30. A 16-year-old man has moderate learning disability and epilepsy. He has a long face with large ears and has hyperextensible joints in his fingers. He is anxious in company and has few friends and a rigid style of communicating.

Multidisciplinary teams

For each patient, choose the *single* most useful member of the multidisciplinary team from the list of options below. Each option may be used once, more than once, or not at all. ★ ★ ★

A Benefits adviser

B Community psychiatric nurse

C Consultant psychiatrist

D Occupational therapist

E Physiotherapist

F Psychologist

G Social worker

H Specialty registrar psychiatrist

I Staff nurse

J Support worker

31. A 26-year-old woman has recently been diagnosed with paranoid schizophrenia after several admissions to hospital. She has been discharged, but there is concern that she does not fully understand or accept the implications of her diagnosis and may stop taking her medication. She needs regular support and education about her illness and relapse prevention.

32. A 37-year-old man with paranoid schizophrenia has been admitted to a rehabilitation ward. His positive symptoms are well controlled with the medication he takes, but he has problems with motivation and the activities of daily living. He has particular difficulties in cooking and shopping for himself and in attending to his personal hygiene. He would like some help to learn how to do these things.

33. A 45-year-old father of two children has severe recurrent depressive episodes that have required hospitalization. He is unable to work for long periods of time, but is hopeful that he may return to part-time employment in the future. However, he is running into financial difficulties because he does not receive any financial support and finds application forms complicated.

34. A 35-year-old woman with bipolar affective disorder is singing loudly late into the night and has been seen in the street wearing very few clothes and bright make-up. She is throwing out large pieces of furniture and is trying to give neighbours' children her money and jewellery, saying she wants to 'spread her wealth'. She requires a review of her mental state with a view to possible admission.

35. A 42-year-old man with obsessive–compulsive disorder is worried because his symptoms have worsened recently. He says he is compliant with his medication, but he has recently lost his job. His wife is concerned that he does not seem 'his usual self', and worries that there might be something else going on. He needs a review.

Single Best Answers

1. B ★   OHCS 8th edn → pp350–351

Alcohol withdrawal can cause delirium tremens, which is characterized by florid visual or tactile hallucinations, typically of small creatures. This is relatively common in drinkers who are suddenly admitted to hospital, and a good alcohol history should always be taken to try and prevent withdrawal by using appropriate medication.

2. D ★   OHCS 8th edn → p192

All patients who have a delayed presentation (more than 8h) after paracetamol overdose should have *N*-acetylcysteine started immediately.

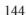

3. E ★

In Munchausen syndrome, or factitious illness, affected people fake illness in order to seek medical attention. Often, reasonably serious symptoms, such as blood in stools or urine, can be falsified. These cannot be reproduced when the person is being directly observed. Malingering is a term used for people who feign illness for another gain, e.g. financial or avoiding work. Hypochondriasis refers to an excessive worry about illness and these patients may often have vague medical symptoms such as palpitations or abdominal pain.

4. C ★   OHCS 8th edn → p362

These are the classical signs of acute opioid intoxication.

5. A ★

The key here is that the person is excessively concerned with an imagined abnormality in physical appearance, which is affecting their life. It is not an obsession and is not affecting mood. The social withdrawal is happening because of the concern about the feature, rather than because of anxiety. Hypochondriasis is a fear of serious illness rather than concern about physical features.

6. D ★   OHCS 8th edn → p363

It is not the amount or quality of what you drink but the effect it has on your life that characterizes dependence.

7. E ★   OHCS 8th edn → p360

Olanzapine is a commonly used atypical antipsychotic. These have fewer side effects than typical antipsychotics, such as haloperidol and chlorpromazine. Lorazepam is a benzodiazepine. Mirtazapine is an antidepressant.

8. C ★   OHCS 8th edn → p340

Depression following MI is associated with poor prognosis, although the evidence that treating depression helps this is equivocal. Tricyclics increase the risk of MI so should not be used in patients with ischaemic heart disease. SSRIs may have a protective effect. Benzodiazepines do not treat depression. MAOIs are used only rarely for depression nowadays due to potentially lethal interactions.

Anon. (2008) Depression, antidepressants and heart disease. *Drug Ther Bull* **46**:29–32.

9. D ★   OHCS 8th edn → p336

Hypothyroidism is a recognized cause of depression and also causes physical symptoms including lethargy, weight gain, constipation, dry skin and hair, and oedema. Recognition of these symptoms should point towards investigating thyroid function to guide appropriate treatment.

10. C ★   OHCS 8th edn → p344

Whilst some of these symptoms may occur in any of the options given, the young age, combination of symptoms and complete resolution in a short time make a panic attack the most likely.

11. B ★   OHCS 8th edn → pp402–403

Although she has signed a consent form, a patient can withdraw consent at any time. Although she has a history of obsessive–compulsive disorder, which would satisfy the definition of a mental disorder under the Mental Health Act 2007 (England and Wales) or the Mental Health (Care and Treatment) (Scotland) Act 2003, she cannot be detained under the Act to allow medical or surgical treatment to continue. The fact that she has pre-eclampsia does not constitute a danger to herself or others (her babies) under the Act, as this risk is not arising from her mental disorder.

12. A ★   OHCS 8th edn → p338

→http://www.medicine.manchester.ac.uk/psychiatry/research/suicide/
prevention/

(Key findings (suicide) from the National Confidential Inquiry into
Suicide and Homicide by People with a Mental Illness)

13. C ★   OHCS 8th edn → p362

A raised MCV and GGT are indicative of problem drinking. Two or more
positive replies are needed on the CAGE questionnaire. Urate levels are
raised in about half of all people with drinking problems, but they are
only useful as screening tests for men as they are poor discriminators
in women. AUDIT is a simple ten-question test developed by the World
Health Organization (WHO) to determine whether a person's alcohol
consumption may be harmful. The test was designed to be used
internationally, and was validated in a study using patients from six
countries. Questions 1–3 deal with alcohol consumption, 4–6 relate to
alcohol dependence, and 7–10 consider alcohol-related problems.
→ http://whqlibdoc.who.int/hq/2001/WHO_MSD_MSB_01.6a.pdf

14. A ★

Cocaine abuse has sympathomimetic effects and causes tachycardia,
hypertension, and pupillary dilatation. Heroin has the opposite effect.
Solvent abuse causes signs similar to alcohol intoxication but may also
include hallucinations. Psilocybin is 'magic mushrooms', which also
causes hallucinations. Oxazepam is a hypnotic drug.

15. C ★

In delirium and in a post-ictal state, there would be alteration in the
level of consciousness. In Alzheimer's disease, the person would have
generalized cognitive impairment that is progressive. Normal pressure
hydrocephalus usually presents with a triad of ataxia, dementia, and
urinary incontinence.

16. C ★   OHCS 8th edn → p403

The Mental Capacity Act 2005 (England and Wales) provides a statutory
framework to empower and protect vulnerable people who are not able
to make their own decisions. It is underpinned by five key principles:

1. Every adult is presumed to have capacity unless it is proven
   otherwise.

2. Individuals must be supported to make their own decisions.

3. Individuals retain the right to make what might be viewed as
   unwise or eccentric decisions.

4. Anything done on behalf of people who lack capacity must be done in their best interests.

5. Anything done on behalf of people who lack capacity must be the least restrictive option.

In this case, the patient has capacity and is not suffering from any mental impairment (e.g. psychotic depression or dementia). Therefore, although it seems an unwise decision, she has the right to refuse surgery. However, in complicated and life-threatening cases such as this, it is always wise to seek a second opinion, and if necessary to involve your trust's legal department. Note that Scotland has a separate legal framework, the Adults with Incapacity (Scotland) Act 2000.

→ http://www.direct.gov.uk/en/DisabledPeople/HealthAndSupport/YourRightsInHealth/DG_10016888
→ http://www.scotland.gov.uk/Publications/2003/03/16933/21228

17. C ★   OHCS 8th edn → p346

An obsession is a stereotyped, purposeless word, idea, or phrase that comes into the mind and that originates from the person, rather than from outside. The patient realizes they are not true.

18. C ★

Bradypnoea, bradycardia, and pin-point pupils strongly suggest opioid overdose. The treatment for this is intramuscular and intravenous naloxone.

19. E ★   OHCS 8th edn → pp350–351, 648, 650

The history of strokes, coupled with the progressive dementia, point to vascular dementia caused by multiple infarcts. Alzheimer's disease is a possibility, but the vascular history suggests otherwise. Lewy body dementia is characterized by hallucinations, visuoperceptual defects, and a fluctuating course. Frontotemporal dementia, or Picks's disease, is characterized by frontal lobe signs such as disinhibition.

20. A ★   OHCS 8th edn → p336

In mild depression, watchful waiting and review is the first strategy. Although this woman has low mood and lack of energy, she is functioning and has no physical symptoms and no suicidal ideation.
→ http://www.nice.org.uk/nicemedia/pdf/CG23quickrefguideamended.pdf (NICE Guideline 23, Depression: Management of Depression in Primary and Secondary Care)

21. B ★   OHCS 8th edn → p344

All could be done, but, as anxiety disorders are maintained by fears about the nature and consequence of symptoms, an explanation of the condition is the first step in treatment. As anxious patients do not concentrate well, especially when given new information, writing down key points so the patient can read them at home is the optimum approach.

22. E ★

Chronic alcohol consumption can result in thiamine deficiency from inadequate nutritional intake, impaired uptake in the bowel, and impaired metabolism. Thiamine deficiency can lead to alcohol-induced brain damage so should be replaced intravenously if patients with alcohol abuse show signs of possible brain damage. The other medications have roles in treating various addictions but are not appropriate in this case.

23. D ★   OHCS 8th edn → p340

All of the others are prominent in tricyclic antidepressants. Confusion is more likely in the elderly prescribed tricyclics, and this together with signs such as dry mouth are due to the anticholinergic effects. Their adrenergic antagonism may cause cardiovascular effects. Citalopram is a selective serotonin reuptake inhibitor (SSRI).

24. B ★   OHCS 8th edn → p360–361

Risperidone is an atypical antipsychotic and is associated with hyperprolactinaemia. This may result in gynaecomastia and galactorrhoea in men, as well as disturbance of the menstrual cycle in women. Risperidone's side effects sometimes include sexual dysfunction and weight gain.

25. E ★ ★

The General Medical Council (GMC) is clear that for several conditions (including dementia) doctors should not only advise patients of the possibility of stopping driving but should also take steps to ensure that the relevant statutory authorities are informed of breaches of regulation if there is reasonable concern about public safety. Initially, this should be done by informing the patient of the need to let the DVLA know about their condition. The fact that the patient is not disorientated, his short-term memory loss is mild and he was only diagnosed a year ago would suggest that you do not have to make an immediate clinical decision that he is unfit to continue driving until the DVLA has assessed him.

Breen D A, Breen D P, Moore J W, Breen P A and O'Neill D (2007) Driving and dementia. *BMJ* **334**:1365–1369.

→http://pb.rcpsych.org/cgi/content/full/25/10/402-a (Royal College of Psychiatrists Public Policy Committee guidance on medical aspects of fitness to drive)

→http://www.gmc-uk.org/guidance/current/library/confidentiality.asp (General Medical Council (2004): Confidentiality: Protecting and Providing Information)

→http://www.dvla.gov.uk/medical/ataglance.aspx/ (Drivers Medical Group. At a glance: current medical standards)

26. E ★★ OHCS 8th edn → p344

There are many different types of anxiety disorder. The fact that all of her symptoms occur in social situations makes social phobia the most likely diagnosis of these.

27. E ★★ OHCS 8th edn → p368

Long-term benzodiazepine use runs the risk of dependency. However, suddenly stopping them may cause a withdrawal syndrome. If this man has run out of diazepam, he risks withdrawal syndrome if he has to wait a week to see his usual GP. Antidepressants will not help the withdrawal. A reducing regime can be used to wean him off the diazepam, but this should be supervised.

28. D ★★ OHCS 8th edn → p354

Lithium has a narrow therapeutic index, meaning that the difference between effective and toxic levels is small. Thirst is a common side effect. Tremor is also common but is fine. Weight gain and skin rash can occur. At toxic levels, dysarthria can occur.

29. E ★★ OHCS 8th edn → p358

Schneider's first-rank symptoms of schizophrenia are symptoms that, if present, are strongly suggestive of schizophrenia. They include:

- Auditory hallucinations: hearing thoughts spoken aloud; hearing voices referring to him- or herself, made in the third person; auditory hallucinations in the form of a commentary

- Thought withdrawal, insertion, and interruption

- Thought broadcasting

- Somatic hallucinations

- Delusional perception

- Feelings or actions experienced as made or influenced by external agents.

30. C ★ ★   OHCS 8ᵗʰ edn → p366

There are a number of personality disorders and each has their own features. They all start in childhood or late adolescence and are patterns of inner experience and behaviour that are stable throughout life and are different from that which would normally be expected in the society in which the person lives. There are two types of emotionally unstable personality disorder: borderline and impulsive. In borderline type. the person tends to form intense relationships and have rapid fluctuations in mood with impulsivity, disturbed self-image, recurrent self-harm, and chronic feelings of emptiness.

31. E ★

Neurosyphilis is an uncommon cause of psychiatric illness but is suggested by the Argyll Robertson pupils as described in the question. They are a highly specific sign of neurosyphilis.

32. D ★

Careful consideration has to be given to team safety when assessing potentially dangerous patients. The police may know the patient and be able to provide valuable information, such as a history of mental health problems or drug use. Additionally, the information the doctor finds out from the police may well influence how and where the patient is seen; for example, it may become clear that the doctor needs to be accompanied by another healthcare professional. The police may well have to leave, and their information should be sought early. Although a quiet, private room may help to calm the patient, it may put the doctor in a dangerous situation. Any room used should be free of potentially dangerous objects and the doctor should always place themselves between the door and the patient. Although having police present for the interview may seem sensible, it will compromise confidentiality, and if the patient has paranoid thoughts or beliefs, a police presence may well increase these. It is better to ask a member of the healthcare staff if there is a need for the doctor to be accompanied.

33. C ★ ★ ★

Under the Mental Capacity Act 2005 (England and Wales), a Personal Welfare LPA does not come into effect *until* the patient has lost capacity to consent, even though it may be registered with the Office of the Public Guardian. As the GP has not seen his patient for 6 months, he does not know whether he has capacity to decide for himself whether to take medication. Although he has a diagnosis of dementia, which may have affected his capacity under the Act, every adult has the right to make his or her own decisions and must be assumed to have capacity to make them unless it is proved otherwise.

Until the GP has assessed the patient, he cannot assume that he does not have capacity. If the GP has assessed the patient and has judged that he does lack capacity to decide to take this medication *and* that prescribing such medication is in his best interests, then the Personal Welfare LPA would allow his wife to give or refuse consent to the carrying out of treatment by a person providing healthcare. Note that a separate act, the Adults with Incapacity (Scotland) Act 2000 is in place in Scotland.

→http://www.publicguardian.gov.uk/index.htm
→http://www.scotland.gov.uk/Topics/Justice/law/awi/helping-friend-relative

34. A ★ ★ ★ ★ OHCS 8th edn → p344

Anxiety management training is a form of cognitive behavioural therapy that has the best record in treatment of anxiety. Behavioural therapy with graded exposure to anxiety-provoking stimuli may be useful in some specific cases. Paroxetine (an SSRI) can help social anxiety, but non-pharmacological measures should be tried first.

35. A ★ ★ ★ ★ OHCS 8th edn → p364

More often than not, a cause cannot be identified, although genetic causes should be considered as they may have implications for genetic counselling. Fragile X syndrome is not X-linked recessive but is caused by an expansion of triplet repeats on the X chromosome through successive generations. Epilepsy can occur in learning disability but only in about 30% of people. There is a spectrum of learning disability and many adults will be able to be supported in finding suitable employment. In mild learning disability, the expected IQ is approximately 50–70, and is 35–50 in moderate learning disability and 20–35 in severe learning disability. However, IQ indicates nothing about individual strengths and weaknesses, so is not the best way of classifying learning disability.

36. B ★ ★ ★ ★ OHCS 8th edn → p394

These are all features suggesting a diagnosis on the autistic spectrum. Autism is a pervasive developmental disorder with features including:

- Impaired communication: at the most severe no language at all, no imaginative play, and echolalia (repeating other people's words)

- Impaired social interaction, e.g. not responding to other people's emotions

- Restricted, repetitive, and stereotyped patterns of movement and behaviours and interests, e.g. liking rigid routines and becoming upset when these do not happen; liking activities such as lining toys up or spinning wheels repeatedly

• Onset before the age of 3 years.

Asperger's syndrome is classified by some as being at one end of the spectrum, but in Asperger's, language is retained although it is qualitatively different. Rett's syndrome occurs in girls.

37. B ★ ★ ★ ★ OHCS 8th edn → p360

There is published guidance in England and Wales on the use of clozapine in the treatment of resistant schizophrenia:
→ http://guidance.nice.org.uk/TA43

38. C ★ ★ ★ ★

If antidepressants are stopped too soon, about 50% of patients relapse. Antidepressants should also be withdrawn over a few weeks.
→ http://www.nice.org.uk/nicemedia/pdf/CG23quickrefguideamended.pdf (NICE Guideline 23, Depression: Management of Depression in Primary and Secondary Care)

39. C ★ ★ ★ ★ OHCS 8th edn → p359

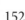

You should familiarize yourself with your local trust's rapid tranquillization policy for cases such as this. In general, start with simple de-escalation techniques (talking calmly, non-hostile body language, etc.), and if necessary offer oral medication first, only moving on to intramuscular administration if the patient refuses. A benzodiazepine such as lorazepam is a good starting point, and you should review the situation regularly. If it is not effective, an antipsychotic should be prescribed. First-generation antipsychotics such as haloperidol are no longer the first choice because of the risk of dystonic side effects. Olanzapine would be an appropriate choice, but note that it cannot be given within an hour of lorazepam.

40. D ★ ★ ★ ★

In the interests of safeguarding children, concerns like this should not be ignored. Good medical practice says that all doctors have a duty to consider the interests of children who may be in the care of adult patients. There are local systems in place to discuss non-urgent concerns, and all trusts will have a designated lead for child protection.
→ http://www.everychildmatters.gov.uk/socialcare/safeguarding/workingtogether/

41. C ★★★★ OHCS 8ᵗʰ edn → p340

Fluoxetine, paroxetine, sertraline, and citalopram are all SSRIs. In situations where patients do not tolerate SSRIs, the next choice would be mirtazapine, a reuptake inhibitor and receptor blocker that affects the levels of noradrenaline (norepinephrine) and serotonin in the synapses.

→ http://www.nice.org.uk/nicemedia/pdf/CG23quickrefguideamended. pdf (NICE Guideline 23, Depression: Management of Depression in Primary and Secondary Care)

42. B ★★★★ OHCS 8ᵗʰ edn → p400

The Mental Health Act 2007 applies to England and Wales. Scotland has a separate Act: the Mental Health (Care & Treatment) (Scotland) Act 2003.

- Section 2 is a (maximum) 28-day section for assessment of someone with a mental disorder. It is used if the diagnosis is not clear.

- Section 3 is a (maximum) 6-month section for treatment. It is only used if the patient is well known and the symptoms fit with the type that he or she suffers from when unwell.

- Section 5 is an emergency holding power, used by nurses (section 5(4)), or doctors (section 5(2)), to detain an informal patient who is already an inpatient.

- Section 17 is the part of the Mental Health Act that allows the Responsible Clinician to grant a detained inpatient leave from the hospital.

- Section 136 is an emergency section used by police to bring someone in a public place who they suspect is suffering from a mental disorder to a place of safety in order that they may be assessed.

→http://www.scotland.gov.uk/Publications/2008/09/24090333/1 (Definitions of terms used in the Mental Health (Care & Treatment) (Scotland) Act 2003)

43. D ★★★★ OHCS 8ᵗʰ edn → p354

→http://www.bnf.org (Registration required)

44. D ★★★★ OHCS 8ᵗʰ edn → p362

Opiate withdrawal is unpleasant, but does not result in death in healthy individuals. Symptoms include restlessness, anxiety, insomnia, abdominal pain, nausea, diarrhoea, yawning, and piloerection. Methadone is a long-acting opiate, with a long half-life, which is taken orally once a day and so reduces the 'rush' from injecting heroin. Naltrexone is an opiate antagonist that can be used after completing detoxification, to reduce the risk of relapse.

45. B ★ ★ ★ ★ OHCS 8th edn → p340

Tricyclic antidepressants can slow cardiac conduction and may cause arrhythmias and heart block. This is particularly dangerous in the elderly, where there may also be a problem with the side effect of postural hypotension.

Extended Matching Questions

1. I ★

Subdurals commonly occur after head injuries. In alcoholics, the injury need only be quite trivial. A subacute subdural typically presents 3–7 days after the injury and causes a variety of symptoms, including headache, confusion, nausea, and weakness.

2. C ★

Delirium is acute confusion, with onset over hours or days. It is common in the elderly when they are in hospital for a number of reasons. Urinary tract infection, as indicated by the abnormal urinalysis, is a common cause. Delirium tremens refers specifically to delirium caused by withdrawal from alcohol.

3. A ★

This is a rare complication of alcohol withdrawal that develops 12–24h after drinking stops. It comes and goes quickly and is limited to auditory hallucinations, unlike delirium tremens, which lasts longer and often has specific visual hallucinations. Wernicke's encephalopathy is an acute, severe thiamine deficiency in alcoholics that causes confusion, memory loss, ataxia, and nystagmus.

4. J ★

There are many causes of dementia. In patients with risk factors for vascular disease, multi-infarct dementia should be considered. It is caused by multiple infarcts in the brain. These may have been silent strokes, without overt clinical signs.

5. K ★

General feedback on 1–5: OHCS 8th edn → pp350–351

6. D ★

Benzodiazepines are commonly used to help relieve symptoms of alcohol detoxification and prevent life-threatening complications such as seizures. Chlordiazepoxide has a slower onset of action and most seizures occur within 48h of stopping alcohol, so diazepam is used where complications are expected. Diazepam should be given under close supervision. Chlordiazepoxide is the first-line treatment in uncomplicated detox programmes at home.

7. I ★

This man has features of a psychosis, probably secondary to the drug misuse. Olanzapine is an atypical antipsychotic, so causes fewer side effects than typical antipsychotics such as haloperidol.

8. A ★

This drug is thought to reduce the cravings for alcohol by stabilizing the imbalance of neurotransmitters in the brain. Disulfiram can also be used in alcoholics but this works by causing an acute sensitivity to alcohol when the person drinks, and will not alter cravings.

9. C ★

10. H ★

This man has signs of Wernicke's encephalopathy, caused by acute, severe thiamine deficiency in alcoholics.

General feedback on 6–10: OHCS 8ᵗʰ edn → pp363, 513

11. G ★

Whilst mini mental state examination alone should not be used to make diagnoses in isolation, it is the most commonly used screening tool for cognitive function. Scores of 25–30 are essentially normal. Coupled with the isolated memory problem and normal life, this indicates a mild impairment only.

12. E ★

Korsakoff's syndrome is part of a spectrum caused by lack of thiamine in the brain in alcoholics. It causes memory loss, vision changes, incoordination, and hallucinations, to varying degrees. The clues here to distinguish this from other forms of memory impairment are the other signs of alcoholic liver disease. Alcohol abuse should always be considered in memory impairment.

13. A ★

This is an enduring, progressive deficit of memory and cognition. In the early stages, there is amnesia and spatial disorientation, whilst in the later stages the personality deteriorates. There are no neurological abnormalities here and no evidence of other disease, which makes other options less likely.

14. C ★

In the elderly, depression is a common cause of memory and functional impairment and should always be screened for. This woman's low mood and poor responses and the short time period make depression likely.

15. H ★

Parkinson's affects the substantia nigra and reduces the amount of dopamine neurotransmitter, which affects signals to the muscles. The main symptoms are slowness of movement (bradykinesia), stiffness of muscles (rigidity), and tremor.

General feedback on 11–15: OHCS 8th edn → pp350–353

16. C ★

Drug abuse is a common cause of acute psychosis in young people and the effects of drugs should be considered before diagnosing other psychotic disorders.

17. G ★

Depression can also have psychotic symptoms. It is important to screen for and recognize depression, as this will alter management.

18. B ★

Delusions are fixed, false beliefs. They can occur as part of schizophrenia, but other symptoms would also need to be present. This man has an isolated delusion.

19. D ★

This is characterized by impulsive behaviour and lack of self-control, along with disturbances of self-image, unstable relationships, feelings of emptiness, and recurrent self-harm. This woman is not hearing voices outside herself, which means that these are not auditory hallucinations seen in psychosis.

20. I ★

This man has hallucinations, delusions, and thought broadcasting that have been evident for more than 6 months.

General feedback on 15–20: OHCS 8th edn → pp356–358

21. F ★ ★

Panic has physical and psychological symptoms. These are typical of the physical symptoms and are affecting her psychologically. Panic disorder is characterized by recurrent, severe panic attacks and behavioural change associated with these. Thinking about the attacks may bring one on.

22. D ★ ★

Generalized anxiety disorder is characterized by excessive, uncontrollable, and often irrational worry about everyday things in a disproportionate way. It interferes with the activities of daily living.

23. B ★ ★

This is a specific panic disorder where the fear is of having a panic attack in a public place. Because of this fear, patients do not leave the house alone. Unfamiliar environments, open spaces, or crowds may be the trigger.

24. H ★ ★

The clear history of a traumatic event here is the clue. In post-traumatic stress disorder, there is an ongoing reaction to the psychological trauma and symptoms such as flashbacks, nightmares, and hyperarousal.

25. J ★ ★

These anxiety symptoms are specific to social situations.

General feedback on 20–25: OHCS 8th edn → pp344–346

26. H ★ ★

Rett's syndrome is X-linked dominant, so only affects girls. There is typically a history of developmental regression, i.e. loss of skills. One of the characteristic movements seen in Rett's is repetitive hand movements. It is the second most common cause of severe learning disability in girls. Genetic testing can be done.

27. A ★★

This is caused by a deletion in the maternally inherited chromosome 15 (deletion on the paternally inherited chromosome 15 causes Prader–Willi syndrome). Children with Angelman's syndrome have characteristic jerky movements and hand flapping, which led to the old-fashioned term 'happy puppet syndrome'. They also have severe epilepsy that can be hard to control. Genetic testing can be done.

28. B ★★

Down's syndrome is now usually diagnosed at birth or at least within the first year of life. However, some older patients may not have had a diagnosis made and are recognized by the characteristic dysmorphic features such as short stature and facial and hand features. There are varying degrees of learning disability in Down's syndrome and many patients can live semi-independently. As people with Down's syndrome get older, they are at high risk of Alzheimer's disease, which usually starts in their 30s.

29. C ★★

The severity of this depends on the level of alcohol consumption in pregnancy. There may not be a clear history of alcohol consumption. Babies are usually small for dates and have microcephaly, as alcohol affects brain development. They have characteristic facial features, which may be subtle, including a hypoplastic upper lip with an absent philtrum (groove) and small eyes with a short palpebral fissure. They have global developmental delay and learning disabilities.

30. D ★★

Fragile X syndrome describes a pattern of inheritance on the X chromosome with triplet repeats that lengthen as they are transmitted from generation to generation. At a critical size, the repeats become unstable and cause problems. Girls and boys can be affected, but boys more severely so because of the lack of another X chromosome. Often, there is a history of mild learning difficulty in the mother and learning difficulty in other male relatives. Boys with fragile X syndrome have characteristic features including large ears and facial asymmetry, and may be on the autistic spectrum. It is the commonest inherited form of learning disability.

General feedback on 26–30: OHCS 8th edn → pp138, 352, 648

31. B ★ ★ ★

Many patients need ongoing support after discharge and it is vital to consider this and to make sure that adequate team support is in place. The role of the community psychiatric nurse is to be a point of contact in the community, support patients through difficult times, support family, help with medication, and check that patients remain well.

32. D ★ ★ ★

An occupational therapist is skilled in assessing how illness impacts on daily life and helps ensure that patients can undertake all of the activities of daily living.

33. A ★ ★ ★

Mental illness can seriously impact on financial well-being for the patient and the whole family, and patients often are unaware of the financial support they may be entitled to. A benefits adviser can help with accessing benefits and filling in forms.

34. C ★ ★ ★

The consultant psychiatrist is best placed to facilitate admission and liaise with all necessary team members. This woman may need admission under the Mental Health Act, so an approved psychiatrist is needed to facilitate this.

35. H ★ ★ ★

The trainee is also a vital member of the team and can see patients on the wards and in clinics.

General feedback on 30–35: → http://www.netdoctor.co.uk/diseases/depression/mentalhealthprofessionals_000358.htm

CHAPTER 4
OPHTHALMOLOGY

Venki Sundaram

Ophthalmology principally aims to prevent visual loss, restore visual function, and relieve ocular discomfort. Ophthalmology is relatively unique in that the majority of the pathology can be directly visualized, therefore requiring proficient ocular examining techniques and visual recognition skills.

Another distinguishing aspect of ophthalmology is the overlap of both medical and surgical conditions. Common systemic diseases such as diabetes and hypertension have ocular features, and diseases involving every organ of the body can have ocular manifestations, so a good depth of medical knowledge is paramount, as well as collaboration with other medical teams. Intraocular surgery for conditions such as cataract is technically challenging, as ocular tissues are so delicate. Therefore, it requires high levels of fine hand–eye co-ordination.

As an ophthalmologist, you will be faced with both acute eye conditions, some of which are sight-threatening and require prompt diagnosis and management, and chronic conditions, which involve monitoring and treatment for many years. You will be exposed to patients of all ages, from premature babies to young children and adults, so good communication with a wide range of patient groups and their families is essential. Patients often say that what they fear most is losing their sight; therefore, empathy and support for patients with debilitating visual impairment is imperative.

The questions in this chapter will test knowledge of acute emergency ophthalmic presentations and the understanding and interpretation of ophthalmic examination, as well as ocular conditions that have systemic associations. In addition, questions relating to ophthalmic risk factors, communication, and probity are given. Eye problems can be daunting to many medical students and doctors. Through practice of examining patients and recognizing key conditions, confidence can be gained in how best to manage these patients and, importantly, when to refer to other specialities. ■

SINGLE BEST ANSWERS

1. A 72-year-old man has painless, sudden of loss of vision in his right eye. Twenty-four hours later, visual acuity in his right eye is counting fingers and there is a carotid bruit on the right side. His blood pressure is 155/100mmHg. His fundus appearance is shown in Plate 4.1. Which is the single most likely diagnosis? ★

A Central retinal artery occlusion

B Central retinal vein occlusion

C Papilloedema

D Rhegmatogenous retinal detachment

E Transient ischaemic attack

2. A 69-year-old hypermetropic woman has had increasing left ocular pain, redness, and blurring of vision for 6h. She is seeing haloes around bright lights. She feels nauseous. Her left eye is shown in Plate 4.2. Which is the single most likely diagnosis? ★

A Acute angle-closure

B Anterior scleritis

C Bacterial conjunctivitis

D Iritis

E Subconjunctival haemorrhage

3. A 72-year-old woman has sudden loss of vision in her right eye. She has been experiencing temporal headache, jaw ache, and shoulder pain for the last 2 weeks. Her visual acuity in the right eye is hand movements. The appearance of her fundus is shown in Plate 4.3. Which single investigation would be most likely to support the diagnosis? ★

A Blood cultures

B CT scan of the head

C Erythrocyte sedimentation rate

D Full blood

E Fluorescein angiography

4. A 54-year-old woman has had increasing, severe right ocular pain for 3 days, which is now affecting her sleep. Her vision is unaffected but she has considerable ocular tenderness. Her right eye is shown in Plate 4.4. Which single systemic condition is most commonly associated with her ocular condition? ★

A Acute lymphocytic leukaemia

B Bacterial endocarditis

C Multiple sclerosis

D Malignant carcinoma of the colon

E Rheumatoid arthritis

5. A 6-year-old boy has had increasing fever, malaise, and right lid swelling over the last 48h. His eyelid is shown in Plate 4.5. When opened with difficulty, he has conjunctival chemosis and mild proptosis, with limitation of upgaze. His temperature is 38.6°C. Which is the single most appropriate treatment? ★

A Intravenous broad-spectrum antibiotics

B Oral antihistamines

C Oral broad-spectrum antibiotics

D Systemic steroids

E Topical antibiotics

6. A 22-year-old man is hit in his right eye with a glass bottle. His vision is 6/24 unaided and his eye is shown in Plate 4.6. Which is the single most serious complication of this injury? ★

A Cataract

B Endophthalmitis

C Hyphaema

D Iridodialysis

E Lens subluxation

7. A 27-year-old woman has accidentally splashed an alkali detergent in both eyes. She is in considerable discomfort and has marked, diffuse bilateral conjunctival injection and hazy corneas. Which is the single most appropriate immediate management? ★

A Application of eye pads

B Irrigation with normal saline

C Limbal stem cell transplant

D Topical antibiotic

E Topical vitamin C

8. A 33-year-old man has had increasing diplopia, drooping of the left upper lid, and headache over the last 2 days. There is a complete left ptosis and the left pupil is dilated. The left eye is depressed and abducted, and eye movements are limited in all directions except downgaze and abduction. Which single condition must be investigated for immediately? ★

A Aponeurotic ptosis

B Myasthenia gravis

C Orbital myositis

D Posterior communicating artery aneurysm

E Thyroid eye disease

9. A 77-year-old woman had uneventful right cataract surgery 3 days ago. She now has increasing pain, redness, and reduced vision in this eye. Vision is 6/60 and there is marked conjunctival injection and anterior chamber inflammation with a 1mm hypopyon. The fundal view is hazy. Which is the single most likely diagnosis? ★

A Acute angle-closure glaucoma

B Bacterial conjunctivitis

C Bacterial endophthalmitis

D Iritis

E Scleritis

10. A 66-year-old man who smokes 15 cigarettes a day has unequal pupil size. Visual acuity is unaffected and his right pupil is smaller, becoming more apparent in darker conditions. His pupils react normally to light and there is mild right upper lid ptosis. Which is the single most appropriate test to confirm the diagnosis of his pupil abnormality? ★ ★

A Chest X-ray

B Erythrocyte sedimentation rate

C MRI scan of the head

D Topical cocaine eye drops

E Topical phenylephrine eye drops

11. A 47-year-old man is referred after being found by his optician on annual check-up to have raised intraocular pressures. He has type 2 diabetes and his uncle is on treatment for glaucoma. Visual acuity is 6/6 in both eyes with glasses for myopia, and intraocular pressures are 34mmHg in the right eye and 36mmHg in the left eye. Which single risk factor is most important for the development of glaucoma? ★ ★

A Age

B Diabetes

C Family history of glaucoma

D Myopia

E Raised intraocular pressure level

12. A 41-year-old woman has had gradual visual loss in her left eye over the last few years. Her optician initially commented that she had an early cataract that was too 'immature' to consider surgery, but this has now progressed. Visual acuity is 6/60 in the left eye and 6/6 in the right. There is a mild left cortical cataract and fundal examination reveals a total rhegmatogenous retinal detachment. Which is the single most appropriate course of action? ★ ★

A Explain in detail the pathological processes involved in developing a retinal detachment

B Explain that she has developed a retinal detachment and discuss the surgical options to reattach the retina and the likely visual prognosis

C Explore why she didn't suspect something more serious was causing her visual loss

D Recommend that she pursues legal action against her optician for delay in diagnosis of a retinal detachment

E Tell her she has a retinal detachment and is likely to go blind in the left eye, but that she still has her other eye

13. A 68-year-old woman with hypertension has gradual decreased vision in her left eye. Her visual acuity is 6/36, improving to 6/9 with pinhole testing, in this eye. Which is the single most likely diagnosis? ★ ★ ★

A Cataract

B Central retinal artery occlusion

C Central retinal vein occlusion

D Dry age-related degeneration

E Glaucoma

14. A 65-year-old woman with multiple sclerosis has reduced right visual acuity. She has type 2 diabetes and underwent squint surgery to her right eye as a child. Her right visual acuity is 6/36 with glasses and there is no pinhole improvement. A swinging flash light test shows a right relative afferent pupillary defect. Which is the single most likely diagnosis? ★ ★ ★ ★

A Amblyopia

B Background diabetic retinopathy

C Cataract

D Diabetic macular oedema

E Optic neuritis

15. A 73-year-old man had routine right cataract surgery 2 weeks ago. At his post-operative visit, his vision is not as clear as he was expecting. Refraction and review of the operation notes reveal a significant (4 dioptre) refractive error due to the wrong power intraocular lens being inserted during surgery. Which is the single most appropriate course of action? ★ ★ ★ ★

A Advise that things will settle and it can take time for the brain to adjust to the new vision

B Apologize and explain that an error has occurred, and involve a senior colleague who can discuss the various management options

C Apologize and explain that the wrong lens was inserted during the operation because the surgeon was handed the wrong power lens

D Apologize that some natural lens fragments have unfortunately been retained in the eye and that a further operation is needed to remove these and replace the lens

E Don't mention that any error has occurred and advise him to visit his optician who can 'fine tune' his vision

EXTENDED MATCHING QUESTIONS

Causes of visual loss

For each patient below with visual loss, choose the *single* most likely diagnosis from the list of options. Each option may be used once, more than once, or not at all. ★

A Anterior ischaemic optic neuropathy

B Branch retinal vein occlusion

C Cataract

D Central retinal artery occlusion

E Central serous retinopathy

F Choroidal neovascular membrane

G Demyelinating optic neuritis

H Diabetic macular oedema

I Diabetic vitreous haemorrhage

J Dry age-related macular degeneration

K Primary open-angle glaucoma

L Retinal detachment

1. A 31-year-old woman has had increasing visual loss in her right eye over the last 3 days and ocular discomfort on eye movement. She has had several episodes of leg weakness in the last 6 months.

2. A 56-year-old man with type 2 diabetes has a sudden reduction of vision in his left eye. The fundal view is poor with ophthalmoscopy, and B-scan ultrasonography shows no retinal detachment.

3. A 72-year-old woman has had increasing difficulty reading over the last 2 years. She has had previous bilateral cataract surgery, and fundul examination shows bilateral macular drusen, atrophy, and pigmentary changes, with no retinal fluid.

4. A 45-year-old man with type 2 diabetes and myopia has loss of vision in the inferior half of his right visual field. There are retinal flame-shaped haemorrhages with vessel tortuosity along the superior vascular arcade.

5. A 67-year-old man has had worsening of central vision in his right eye over the last week. There is a submacular greyish lesion on the fundus with subretinal oedema and haemorrhage.

ANSWERS

Single Best Answers

1. A ★   OHCS 8th edn → p435

A pale fundus with a 'cherry-red' spot at the macula is classically found in central retinal artery occlusions. Hypertension and sources of potential emboli (e.g. carotid artery disease) are risk factors for developing this condition.

2. A ★   OHCS 8th edn → p430

Ocular pain and nausea are due to the acute rise in intraocular pressure. This also causes corneal oedema with reduced vision and glare symptoms. Examination findings are typically ciliary vessel injection, mid-dilated pupil, shallow anterior chamber depth, and high intraocular pressure (>40mmHg). Increasing age and hypermetropia are risk factors for developing acute angle-closure.

3. C ★   OHCS 8th edn → p434

This woman has a left anterior ischaemic optic neuropathy, secondary to giant cell arteritis (temporal arteritis). A very raised erythrocyte sedimentation rate is typically found, and patients can experience temporal headache, jaw pain, and myalgia. The posterior ciliary arteries may be affected by the arteritis, resulting in an anterior ischaemic optic neuropathy causing dramatic visual loss and a swollen disc with flame-shaped haemorrhages.

4. E ★   OHCS 8th edn → p448

This woman has a right diffuse anterior scleritis. This is associated with an underlying autoimmune condition in nearly 50% of cases, of which rheumatoid arthritis is the most common.

5. A ★   OHCS 8th edn → p420

This boy has a right-sided orbital cellulitis, which usually arises from bacterial spread from adjacent sinuses. This differs from preseptal cellulitis, as congestion from orbital spread results in chemosis, proptosis, and restriction of eye movement, in addition to just eyelid involvement. This is an emergency, requiring urgent intravenous antibiotics and possible drainage of any sinus abscess. A delay in treatment can result in complications such as optic nerve compression and meningeal spread.

6. B ★   OHCS 8ᵗʰ edn → p452

This man has a penetrating eye injury. This requires urgent closure of the corneoscleral laceration, with appropriate antibiotic cover. A delay in management can increase the risk of developing endophthalmitis and can result in severe, permanent visual loss.

7. B ★   OHCS 8ᵗʰ edn → p452

Alkali eye injuries are potentially sight-threatening, as they can cause liquefactive necrosis of ocular tissue. Immediate copious irrigation with normal saline until a neutral pH is reached can prevent further alkali penetration and destruction.

8. D ★

This man has a left-sided third-nerve palsy. Pupil involvement implies a compressive cause, and the rapid, painful onset suggests an expanding lesion such as a posterior communicating artery aneurysm. This needs to be investigated immediately to prevent a potentially fatal subarachnoid haemorrhage.

9. C ★   OHCS 8ᵗʰ edn → p442

Post-operative bacterial endophthalmitis is a rare but serious complication of cataract surgery. Patients typically present with poor vision, pain, and significant intraocular inflammation within 2 weeks of surgery. The fundal view can be obscured by significant vitritis. Prompt recognition and management can help prevent irreversible visual loss.

10. D ★ ★   OHCS 8ᵗʰ edn → p424

This man has right-sided Horner's syndrome. This occurs because of interrupted sympathetic innervation to the eye. Topical 4% cocaine drops instilled into both eyes will only cause dilatation of the normal pupil. This is because cocaine blocks the reuptake of noradrenaline (norepinephrine) at nerve endings, causing pupil dilatation. In Horner's syndrome, no noradrenaline is secreted so cocaine has no effect. Horner's syndrome can occur with Pancoast tumours of the lung, as well as other causes.

11. E ★ ★   OHCS 8ᵗʰ edn → p440

Raised intraocular pressure is the strongest risk factor for the development and progression of glaucoma. Lowering of intraocular pressure is currently the only method of preventing visual field loss.

12. B ★ ★

The news that this woman's visual loss is from a retinal detachment rather than cataract is likely to come as a shock and be anxiety-provoking. Therefore, this needs to be conveyed in a sensitive manner without blame on her or other professionals. Focus can then be given to the management options available, including what possible surgery would involve and the likely visual outcome.

13. A ★ ★ ★   OHCS 8th edn → p442

Pinhole use focuses light entering the eye, so can compensate for refractive errors (up to several dioptres) or conditions that cause glare, such as cataract. Visual acuity improvement with pinhole testing therefore implies a refractive problem, rather than an organic problem.

14. E ★ ★ ★ ★   OHCS 8th edn → p434

A relative afferent pupillary defect occurs when light shone into the affected eye causes initial dilatation of both pupils. The pupils initially dilate because the stimulus from light being shone into the affected eye is less than the stimulus of withdrawing light from the unaffected eye. This most commonly occurs in optic nerve lesions, but can also be due to other gross pathology of the anterior visual pathway (e.g. total retinal detachment, optic tract lesions).

15. B ★ ★ ★ ★

For a variety of reasons, insertion of the wrong power intraocular lens during cataract surgery unfortunately occurs. Patients have a right to know and need to be appropriately informed of such errors and the various management options, so that they can make an informed decision on how best to rectify any visual difficulties.

The surgeon carrying out the operation is ultimately responsible for the power of the intraocular lens inserted, even if handed the wrong one by a scrub nurse or assistant.

Careful pre-operative selection, double-checking of the correct lens power, and the surgeon themselves obtaining the correct lens from the lens storage can help ensure that the correct lens is inserted.

Extended Matching Questions

1. G ★

Multiple sclerosis is a disease of demyelination that can affect the optic nerve and cause optic neuritis. The distinct episodes of weakness are caused by demyelination of peripheral nerves.

2. I ★

Sudden reduction of vision with a poor fundal view in diabetic patients implies a vitreous haemorrhage from proliferative diabetic retinopathy. B-scan ultrasonography can be useful in excluding large retinal tears or detachment as the cause of the vitreous haemorrhage.

3. J ★

Gradual visual loss (especially difficulty with reading) is typical of dry age-related macular degeneration. Both eyes are usually affected, with macular drusen, atrophy, and retinal pigment epithelial changes seen.

4. B ★

This produces haemorrhage and vessel tortuosity in the region of the affected vessel. This can cause corresponding visual field loss (i.e. inferior field loss in superior occlusions) as retinal images are inverted.

5. F ★

Choroidal neovascular membranes can appear as greyish lesions beneath the macula. Leakage of blood or fluid from the membrane usually results in fairly acute onset of central visual loss due to photoreceptor damage.

General feedback on 1–5: OHCS 8th edn →pp434–439

CHAPTER 5
PRIMARY CARE

Will Coppola and Kamila Hawthorne

GPs are the gatekeepers of the National Health Service in the UK, and virtually all referrals to secondary care are made through them. The breadth and depth of the discipline can, at times, seem overwhelming, although the old adage 'common things occur commonly' still holds. GPs need to be confident in the diagnosis and management of conditions from birth to the grave, and to know their boundaries of competence and when to refer to secondary care. The complexity of the GP consultation includes the following points:

1) Many conditions present in a relatively undifferentiated form to the GP, whose job it is to try to identify whether it is normal or abnormal, serious or minor.

2) GPs develop a close professional relationship with many of their patients and may also be the point of contact for other members of the family, neighbours, and friends of the patient. This knowledge is an important aspect of their holistic approach to medicine, and is much valued by their patients. As the 19th-century physician Sir William Osler (1849–1919) said, '*The good physician treats the disease; the great physician treats the patient who has the disease*'.

The commonest presentations to GPs in the UK are for respiratory problems, chronic disease management, musculoskeletal and psychological problems. Health promotion, in particular smoking cessation and the management of obesity, is also important in preventing chronic illness. Although many presentations are minor and self-limiting, serious illnesses also occur and GPs need to be able to recognize them, sometimes at early stages.

The questions in this chapter will assess in the common areas that present, testing diagnostic skills and reasoning. They also test negotiating skills to ensure patient compliance, team working within the primary care setting, and risk management. ■

Kamila Hawthorne

PRIMARY CARE
SINGLE BEST ANSWERS

1. A 26-year-old woman has registered as a new patient and her new-patient health check reveals a body mass index (BMI) of 32 kg/m². Which is the single best explanation to the patient of what BMI means? ★

A It is a measure of cardiovascular risk

B It is a measure of how much weight a person needs to lose

C It is a representation of weight for height

D It is a way of calculating how fat the body is

E It is the ratio of hip circumference to waist circumference

2. A 44-year-old builder has acute low back pain following heavy lifting at work the previous day. He is finding it difficult to walk. Which single feature of his presentation would warrant urgent referral to hospital? ★

A Difficulty passing urine

B Inability to perform a straight leg raise beyond 20°

C Pain down the back of both legs

D Reduced ankle jerks

E Use of inhaled steroids for his asthma

3. The mother of a 16-year-old girl is worried that her daughter is becoming depressed and she knows the girl came to see you last week. The daughter's behaviour has been deteriorating at home and there have been a lot of arguments. She wants to know what that consultation was about and to get your opinion about what to do. Which is the single most appropriate course of action? ★

A Advise her that she can apply to the primary care trust for access to her daughter's medical record

B Do not discuss her concerns about her daughter at all as the daughter is over 16 years of age

C Listen to her concerns but do not reveal information about the daughter as the daughter has not given you consent

D Tell her a little bit about the consultation and ask her to come back later with her daughter

E Tell her what transpired in the recent consultation as she has a right to know as a parent

4. A 65-year-old man has had a previous small myocardial infarction. He wants advice on modifying his risk factors to prevent further health problems. Which is the single most important modifiable risk factor for stroke for this patient? ★

A Alcohol intake of 40 units per week

B Atrial fibrillation

C Body mass index of 35kg/m²

D Previous myocardial infarction

E Raised blood pressure of 165/105 mmHg

5. A 44-year-old business man has recently been diagnosed with high blood pressure. He does not want to take medication. Which is the single best approach to take in the consultation to try and come to a resolution? ★

A Allow him to do what he wants to do, but tell him he has to see another doctor in the future

B Be friendly towards him, so he is more likely to come back if he changes his mind

C Identify and consider his viewpoint, bringing this into the decision-making process

D Tell him all about the different medications and their side effects so he has all the information

E Tell him he needs to take the medication chosen for him or he may be at risk of harm

6. A 35-year-old woman is unable to sleep, is tired during the day, and is having problems at work as a result. Which single aspect of her history is the most likely to have a significant bearing on her presenting complaint? ★

A She drinks about 20 units of alcohol per week

B She has a 9-year-old daughter

C She has a stressful job as a teacher

D She is tearful and cannot concentrate

E She smokes ten cigarettes a day

7. A 17-year-old girl is going away to college next year. She is seeking information about the human papilloma virus (HPV) vaccine as she is considering having it. Which is the single most appropriate piece of information to give her about the vaccine? ★

A If she has already had sexual intercourse, she has probably already been exposed to HPV and it is not worth having the vaccination

B If she has the vaccination, it will protect her against getting HPV and she will not need cervical smear testing later in life

C If she suffers from eczema or asthma, she will not be able to have the vaccination for fear of severe allergic reactions

D The vaccination is only available as part of a primary immunization course for infants and she is too old to be in the 'catch-up' cohort

E The vaccination is 99% effective in preventing cervical abnormalities caused by HPV types that can lead to cervical cancer and she is eligible to have it

8. A 52-year-old woman wants advice about mammography breast screening before her appointment. She has read a newspaper article that suggests that it may not be valuable and could even be potentially harmful. You are not aware of this evidence and have not seen any recent literature on the subject. Which is the single most appropriate response to give in this situation? ★

A Advise her that there is a financial penalty for practices if patients do not attend screening appointments so she should make every effort to go

B Agree with her that there are reasonable concerns about the benefits of mammography and advise her not to take any further part in the screening programme

C Explain that you are not aware of the evidence that she has raised with you so you are going to refer her to a specialist breast surgeon for up-to-date advice

D Explain that you are not aware of the evidence that she has raised with you, but that you could help her interpret it once you have looked at it yourself

E Explain that you are not aware of the evidence that she has raised with you so it is highly unlikely to be true and she should attend

9. A 48-year-old woman has recently moved into the practice area. At her induction health check, the practice nurse notes that her weight is 85kg and her height is 160cm. Which single health factor would you consider in advising her about her weight? ★

A She is at increased risk of stomach cancer and needs to lose weight to a body mass index (BMI) of 25 kg/m² to bring her risk down to acceptable levels

B She is at increased risk of stomach cancer and needs to lose 20kg to bring her risk down to acceptable levels

C She is at increased risk of hypertension and should lose 5kg to bring her risk down to acceptable levels

D She is at increased risk of kidney stones and needs to lose 10kg to bring her risk down to acceptable levels

E She is at increased risk of type 2 diabetes and should lose 20kg to bring her risk down to acceptable levels

10. A 22-year-old student has muscle aches, malaise, headache, and anorexia that started 2 days ago. Today he has a temperature of 39.4°C. Which is the single most important direct question to ask him as part of history-taking in order to confirm the likely diagnosis? ★

A Has he been bitten by an animal recently?

B Has he had close contact with anyone else with similar symptoms?

C Has he recently eaten anything that he thinks might have been off?

D Has he travelled overseas recently?

E Is he taking any medication at present?

11. A 55-year-old diabetic man asks for the vaccines he had last year against flu and pneumonia. His records show he had the influenza and pneumococcal vaccines last year. Which is the single most appropriate piece of advice to give him? ★

A The influenza vaccine he had last year will protect him against influenza for another 5 years

B He does not need another influenza vaccine this year but should have it next year

C He does not need another pneumococcal vaccine this year but should have it next year

D He is in a high-risk category for influenza and should have this vaccine every year

E He is in a high-risk category for pneumonia and influenza and should have both vaccines every year

12. A 50-year-old man with convictions for violence comes to the surgery reception smelling of alcohol and demanding dihydrocodeine. Which is the single best way of managing this situation? ★

A Ask him to take a seat in the waiting room to be seen in order with other patients

B Immediately show him to the next available doctor

C Phone the police and ask them to remove him

D Physically eject him from the premises and lock the surgery door

E Place him in a vacant room and ask a doctor to see him when available

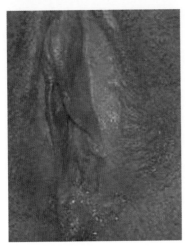

Plate 1.1

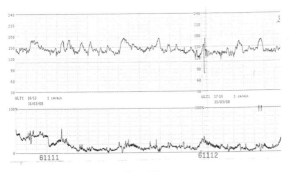

Plate 1.2

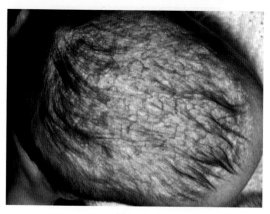

Plate 2.1

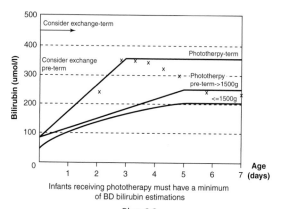

Infants receiving phototherapy must have a minimum
of BD bilirubin estimations

Plate 2.2

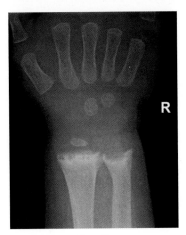

Plate 2.3

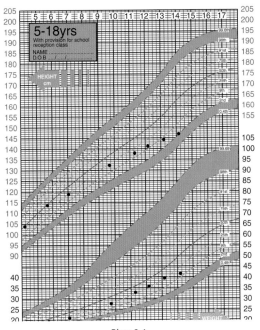

Plate 2.4

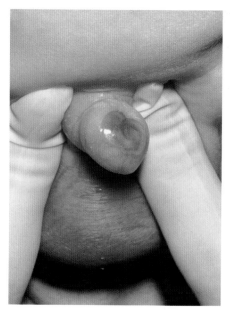

Plate 2.5

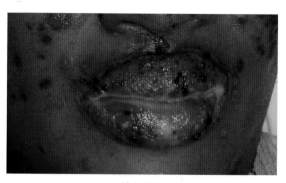

Plate 2.6

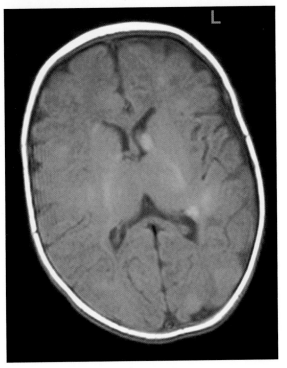

Plate 2.7

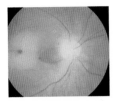

Plate 4.1

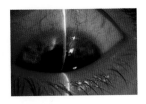

Plate 4.2

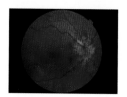

Plate 4.3

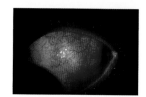

Plate 4.4

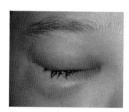

Plate 4.5

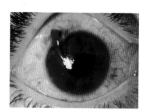

Plate 4.6

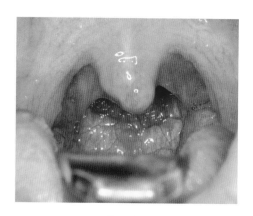

Plate 6.1

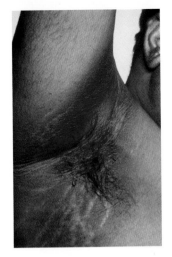

Plate 7.1

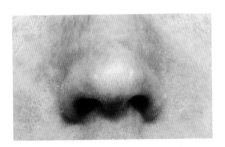

Plate 7.2

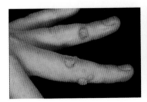

Plate 7.3

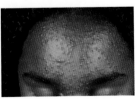

Plate 7.4

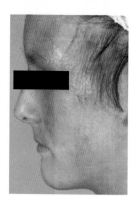

Plate 7.5

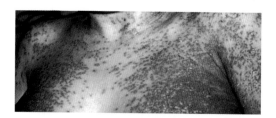

Plate 7.6

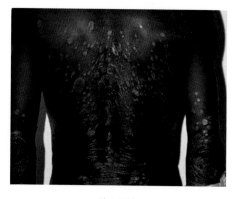

Plate 7.7

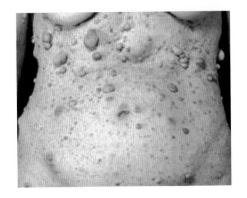

Plate 7.8

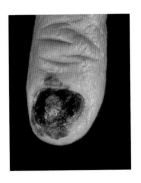

Plate 7.9

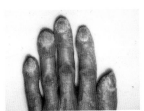

Plate 7.10

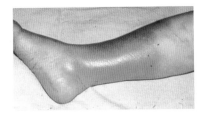

Plate 7.11

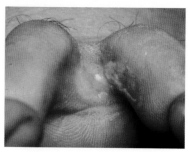

Plate 7.12

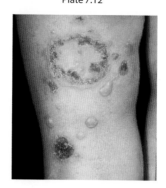

Plate 7.13

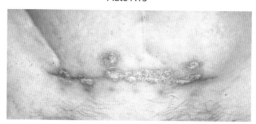

Plate 7.14

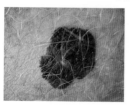

Plate 7.15

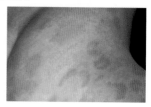

Plate 7.16

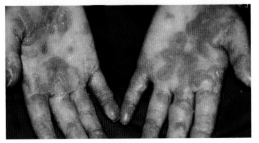

Plate 7.17

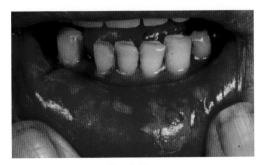

Plate 7.18a

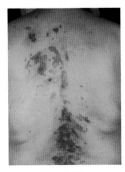

Plate 7.18b

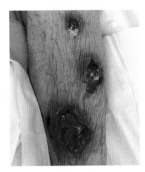

Plate 7.19

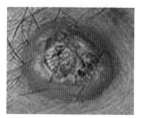

Plate 7.20

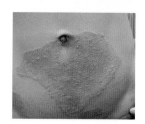

Plate 7.21

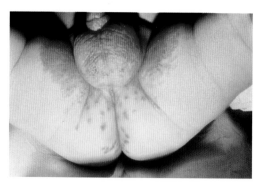

Plate 7.22

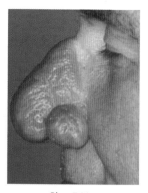

Plate 7.23

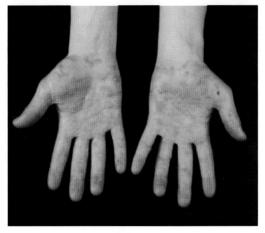

Plate 7.24

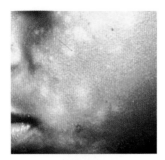

Plate 7.25

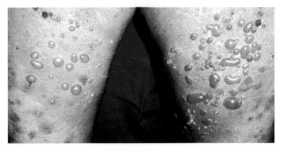

Plate 7.26

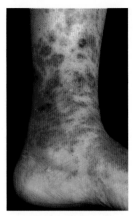

Plate 7.27

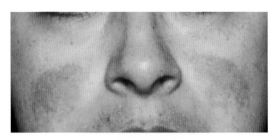

Plate 7.28

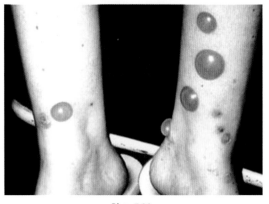

Plate 7.29

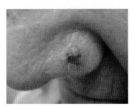

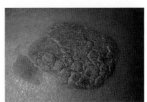

Plate 7.30

Plate 7.31

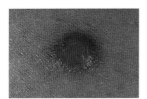

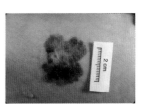

Plate 7.32

Plate 7.33

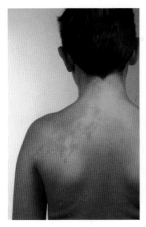

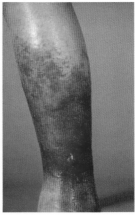

Plate 7.34

Plate 7.35

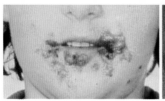

Plate 7.36

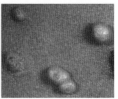

Plate 7.37

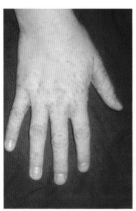

Plate 7.38

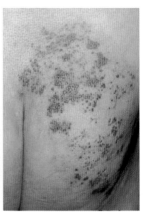

Plate 7.39

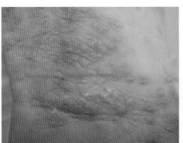

Plate 7.40

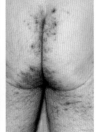

Plate 7.41

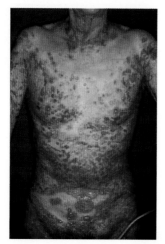

Plate 7.42

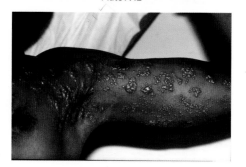

Plate 7.43

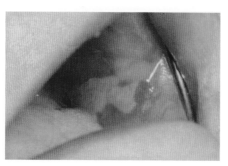

Plate 7.44

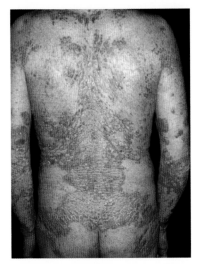

Plate 7.45

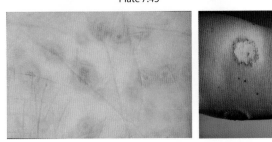

Plate 7.46

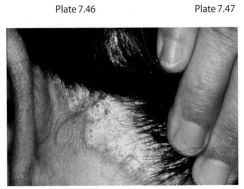

Plate 7.47

Plate 7.48

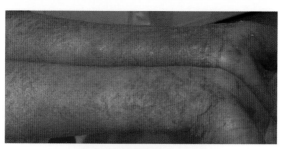

Plate 7.49

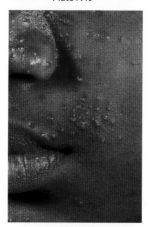

Plate 7.50

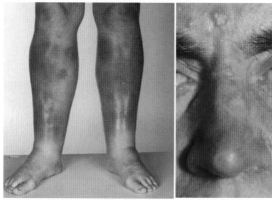

Plate 7.51

Plate 7.52

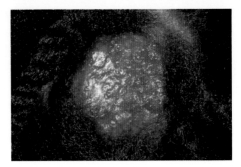

Plate 7.53

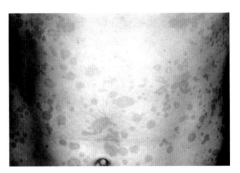

Plate 7.54

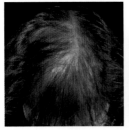

Plate 7.55

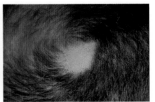

Plate 7.56

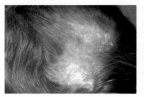

Plate 7.57

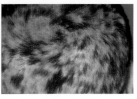

Plate 7.58

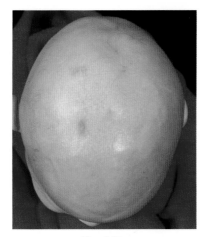

Plate 7.59

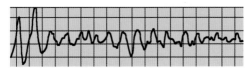

Plate 8.1

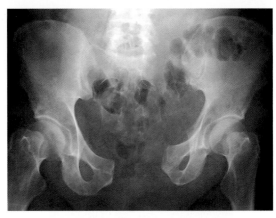

Plate 9.1

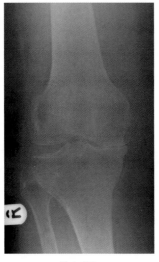

Plate 9.2

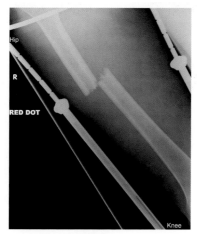

Plate 9.3

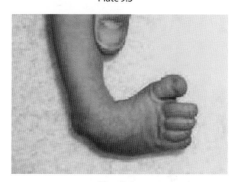

Plate 9.4

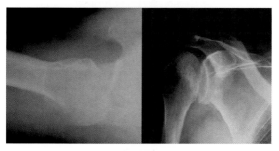

Plate 9.5

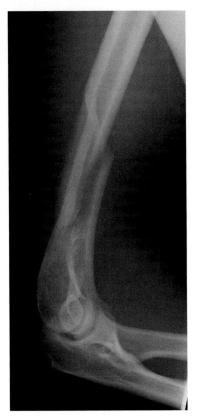

Plate 9.6

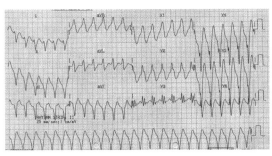

Plate 10.1

13. An 84-year-old woman is in hospital recovering from a total hip replacement following a fall in her flat. She was previously independent, despite living on the first floor, and drove her own car to the nearby shops. Who is the single best professional to ensure that she is safe to return to her flat? ★

A Age Concern worker

B GP

C Health visitor

D Occupational therapist

E Physiotherapist

14. An 18-year-old man has a sore throat, fever, and malaise. A monospot test is sent and comes back positive. Which is the single most important element to avoid at this stage? ★

A Alcohol

B Contact sports

C Fatty foods

D Kissing

E Paracetamol

15. A 21-year-old student comes for a repeat prescription of her combined oral contraceptive pill (the Pill). She has been getting bad one-sided headaches with flashing lights lasting a few minutes prior to the headache since starting the Pill. She has a past history of migraine when stressed and has some exams coming up. Her blood pressure is 100/70mmHg and clinical examination is normal. Which is the single most appropriate management? ★

A Advise her that the headaches are most probably caused by exam stress

B Advise her to stop taking the Pill if the flashing lights last longer than 60 min

C Stop the Pill and try a different combined oral contraceptive pill

D Stop the Pill and consider a progestogen-only pill instead

E Stop the Pill and refer her to a neurologist urgently

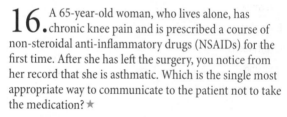

16. A 65-year-old woman, who lives alone, has chronic knee pain and is prescribed a course of non-steroidal anti-inflammatory drugs (NSAIDs) for the first time. After she has left the surgery, you notice from her record that she is asthmatic. Which is the single most appropriate way to communicate to the patient not to take the medication? ★

A Ask the receptionist to make her a routine appointment for the next day

B Phone her and give her the appropriate advice

C Phone the local chemist and instruct them not to issue the prescription

D Phone the police and ask them to go to her house

E Write to her requesting that she make an urgent appointment

17. A 21-year-old single mother has a 2-month-old baby who is not sleeping and seems perpetually hungry. She is still breastfeeding, but thinks she will have to change her baby to bottle-feeding. She wants some advice about this. Who is the single best person from the health-care team to advise her? ★

A District nurse

B GP

C Health visitor

D Midwife

E Social worker

18. A 22-year-old woman has persistent headaches, nausea, and disturbed sleep. She appears very thin and her body mass index (BMI) is $16kg/m^2$. She tells you that this is her normal weight. Which single healthcare professional would it be most appropriate to refer her to? ★

A Counsellor

B Continue to see her yourself as a GP

C Dietician

D Endocrinologist

E Psychiatrist

19. A 32-year-old woman is 33 weeks pregnant with her second child. She has come for a routine antenatal appointment. In her first pregnancy, she suffered pre-eclampsia and required a hospital admission and early delivery. Today she is feeling tired and off-colour. Which single combination of clinical features would suggest that she could be suffering from pre-eclampsia requiring immediate hospital referral? ★

A Raised blood pressure alone

B Raised blood pressure and proteinuria

C Raised blood pressure, proteinuria, and headache

D Raised blood pressure, proteinuria, and peripheral oedema

E Raised blood pressure, proteinuria, and seizures

20. A 17-year-old man has had a sore throat, fever, malaise, and headache for 4 days. He has bilaterally enlarged tonsils with exudate, and cervical lymphadenopathy. Which single complication of his illness can be prevented by treatment with oral penicillin? ★

A Drug eruption

B Glomerulonephritis

C Mesenteric adenitis

D Otitis media

E Sinusitis

21. A 65-year-old woman with osteoarthritis affecting both knees is in need of some pain relief. However, she is unwilling to take anti-inflammatories as she says they make her feel ill and pain killers make her constipated. She asks whether complementary medicine can help her. Which single type of complementary medicine has the most evidence of efficacy? ★ ★

A Aromatherapy with oil of evening primrose.

B Glucosamine and chondroitin

C Homeopathy

D Modern acupuncture using trigger points

E Reflexology

22. A man has a chest infection. He is prescribed a course of amoxicillin for a week. He also wants a repeat prescription of his blood pressure medication. Under which single circumstance is he eligible to get the medications without paying prescription charges for them? ★

A He earns less than £25,000 per annum

B He has a partner and more than three children at home

C He has been unwell for more than 4 weeks

D He has diabetes

E He is aged over 50 years

23. A 35-year-old woman is 12 weeks pregnant. She has significant dysuria, urinary frequency, and offensive-smelling urine. A dipstick test shows 3+ blood, 3+ leukocytes, and 2+ nitrites. Which single regime is the most appropriate treatment? ★ ★

A Amoxicillin for 7 days

B Encourage oral fluids and simple analgesia

C Nalidixic acid for 7 days

D Nitrofurantoin for 7 days

E Trimethoprim for 3 days

24. A 55-year-old man has raised blood pressure. Which is the single most appropriate device to measure his present blood pressure in the GP surgery? ★ ★

A Aneroid sphygmomanometer

B Ambulatory blood pressure monitor

C Automated elbow blood pressure monitor

D Automated wrist blood pressure monitor

E Mercury sphygmomanometer

25. A 50-year-old man seeks advice about his father, who has mild dementia and is living in a nursing home. The father is becoming increasingly unwell with a chest infection and the son wants him to be admitted to hospital, but the father wishes to stay where he is. Which is the single best summary of the legal situation? ★ ★

A As the father has dementia, he is not competent and therefore the son can and should decide on his treatment

B The father is competent and therefore can decide on his own treatment, regardless of the son's opinion

C The father is not competent and therefore decisions about his care must be made by his doctor based on the patient's best interests

D The father's competence should be assessed and, if he has capacity, he is able to accept or decline treatment himself regardless of the consequences

E The father's competence should be assessed, but his doctor may insist on admission, should his condition deteriorate, on the grounds of necessity

26. A 35-year-old woman with persistent irritable bowel syndrome asks to see a complementary therapist to help her with her symptoms. She understands that she may need to pay for this privately and that there may not be good evidence for the effectiveness of some complementary treatments, but she says that she is convinced that this is what she would like. Which is the single most appropriate action to take in response to her request? ★ ★

A Ask her to identify a practitioner she would like to see and then provide a written referral if requested

B Decline to refer her on the grounds that that this will avoid private care fees

C Refer her directly to a colleague who runs a private complementary clinic

D Refer her to a gastroenterologist because she is more likely to achieve better symptom control with a conventional specialist

E Refer her to a therapist selected from the Yellow Pages on the basis of geographical proximity to her home

27. A 65-year-old woman, who regularly attends with symptoms related to chronic depression, has some vague muscle ache and headache. She has been told before that her symptoms may well be related to her depression but requests further assessment. Which single aspect of her history is the most likely to point to a significant alternative diagnosis? ★ ★

A She has been getting pain in her hip when walking

B She has been getting some stinging pain on passing urine

C She has noticed a deterioration of her vision

D She has noticed some hearing loss in her left ear

E She has recently started taking herbal remedies for her depression

28. The local pharmacist has sent back a prescription written this morning. He says that a controlled drug has been prescribed wrongly—a patient with intractable chronic back pain has been given a prescription for morphine modified release (MST Continus®). Which single element must be on a prescription for a controlled drug? ★ ★

A The date must be written in words and figures

B The diagnosis must be specified

C The full name and address of the patient must be handwritten, not typed

D The prescriber's General Medical Council registration number must be given

E The total quantity to dispense must be expressed in words and figures

29. A medical student is sitting in on a GP surgery. One of the patients says he would rather not have a student present. Which is the single most appropriate way of handling this? ★ ★ ★

A Before calling the patient in, ask the student to wait in another room

B Emphasize the importance of student teaching, hoping that the patient will reconsider

C Introduce the student and confirm that the patient would prefer the student to leave

D Rebook the patient for another surgery when you don't have students present

E Reschedule the patient to the end of surgery

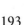

30. A 62-year-old woman has had a unilateral painful rash highly suggestive of shingles for 36h. She asks if she could pass it on to her grandson, aged 7 days. He lives in the same town and she last saw him yesterday. The baby's mother doesn't think she has ever had chickenpox. Which is the single most appropriate piece of advice to give to the grandmother? ★ ★ ★

A As the baby has been in contact, he should receive zoster immunoglobulin (ZIG) as soon as possible

B It is better to get chickenpox while you are a child than later in life, and she need not worry about contact

C It is better to get shingles while you are a child than later in life, and she need not worry about contact

D The baby could get chickenpox and she should avoid seeing him until the blisters crust over

E The baby will be protected by maternal antibodies and will not be affected

EXTENDED MATCHING QUESTIONS

Causes of chest pain

For each patient with acute chest pain, choose the *single* most likely diagnosis from the list of options below. Each option may be used once, more than once, or not at all. ★

A Bornholm's disease

B Costochondritis

C Dissecting aortic aneurysm

D Idiopathic chest pain

E Musculoskeletal chest pain

F Myocardial infarction

G Oesophageal spasm

H Pericarditis

I Pleurisy

J Pneumothorax

K Pulmonary embolus

L Shingles

1. A 63-year-old woman has had severe pain on the right side of her chest, over the right breast, for 2 days. The pain is constant and sharp, and is not affected by taking in a deep breath, coughing, or movement. She has no past medical history of note, is on no regular medication, and is a non-smoker. She is distressed by the pain, but is not sweaty or short of breath. Her pulse rate is 76bpm and her blood pressure is 140/88mmHg. She has some tenderness on the right side of her chest with hyperaesthesia.

2. A 45-year-old man tore his right anterior cruciate ligament 5 days ago while skiing in Canada. It was repaired abroad and he has flown home. He has had sharp central chest pain for the past 8h, which is worse on taking a deep breath. He feels short of breath and is a little sweaty. His respiratory rate is 25/min, his blood pressure is 100/60mmHg, his pulse rate is 100bpm, and there is a pleural rub on the left side of his chest.

3. A 40-year-old woman has had chest pain for the last 4 days. The pain is worse on movement, coughing, or sneezing, and is slightly worse on taking a deep breath in. She feels very tired and has been unable to continue with her usual daily activity – she is a nurse at the local hospital and is married with three children. Her pulse rate is 68bpm and regular, and her blood pressure is 120/82mmHg. She has marked local tenderness to palpation on the left side, over her sternum, with no associated heat, erythema, or swelling.

4. A 55-year-old man has had central chest pain for 2h, radiating to his shoulders. The pain came on gradually over a few minutes while walking his dog, and is a tight pain or discomfort that feels like a pressure on his chest. It is not affected by position or coughing. He feels nauseated and sweaty and is very anxious. He smokes 20 cigarettes a day. He looks clammy and is short of breath. His pulse rate is 88bpm and his blood pressure is 110/60mmHg. His heart sounds are normal and his chest sounds clear.

5. A 38-year-old woman has had a sharp, constant sternal pain for the last 24h, which came on suddenly. Prior to this, she had had a heavy head cold for 5 days. The pain radiates to the left shoulder and is worse if she is lying on her left side. Taking a deep breath, coughing, and swallowing also make it worse. The pain is relieved a little by sitting forward. A scratchy rub can be heard over the left sternal border, which is louder when she leans forwards.

Causes of dizziness

For each patient complaining of dizziness, choose the *single* most likely diagnosis from the list of options below. Each option may be used once, more than once, or not at all. ★

A Benign positional vertigo

B Cardiac arrhythmia

C Cerebellar disorder

D Cough syncope

E Hyperventilation

F Hypoglycaemia

G Ménière's syndrome

H Postural hypotension

I Pre-syncope

J Tumour

K Vertebrobasilar insufficiency

L Viral labyrinthitis

6. A 55-year-old man has type 1 diabetes and has had bouts of severe dizziness, lasting a few minutes each time, for 10 days. His surroundings are spinning and he feels nauseated at the time. It occurs with changes in posture and he has attacks up to ten times a day. It is not related to other activities and he has been eating and checking his capillary blood glucose as normal. He had a viral illness about 2 weeks ago. He has no nystagmus, Romberg's sign is negative, and his ENT examination is normal. He has a positive Hallpike test.

7. A 26-year-old man has type 1 diabetes. He had dizziness, which came on fairly rapidly over a couple of minutes just before lunchtime at work. He had an early start that day, but his capillary blood glucose in the morning had been 7.0mmol/L. He had a similar episode about 3 months earlier, also when at work. He looks clammy and sweaty and generally unwell. His speech is slightly slurred.

8. A 21-year-old man had a sudden onset of vertigo, nausea, and vomiting 36h ago. He is unable to lift his head off the pillow because the room starts to spin. He has no loss of hearing, no tinnitus, and his ENT examination is normal. His pulse rate is 56bpm and his blood pressure is 110/70mmHg.

9. A 50-year-old woman has had dizziness and difficulty walking since she woke up 3 days ago. She has hypertension and is on bendroflumethiazide. She appears intoxicated, with a wide-based gait and slightly slurred speech. She is unable to walk in a straight line. She is unable to perform repetitive movements and has a rotary nystagmus in both eyes.

10. A 35-year-old woman has attacks of recurrent vertigo that started about 8 months ago. Attacks can come on at any time and are associated with nausea and a feeling of fullness in the right ear. They last up to 3–4h. She thinks she may be becoming deaf on that side. Her grandmother had something similar. The tinnitus is driving her mad and stops her from sleeping.

Causes of fever

For each patient with fever, choose the *single* most likely diagnosis from the list of options below. Each option may be used once, more than once, or not at all. ★

A Appendicitis

B *Campylobacter* gastroenteritis

C Cholecystitis

D Hodgkin's lymphoma

E Malaria

F Meningococcal meningitis

G Menopausal flushing

H Pancreatitis

I Pneumonia

J Pyelonephritis

K Subacute bacterial endocarditis

L Tuberculosis

M Viral gastroenteritis

N Viral hepatitis

O Viral upper respiratory tract infection

11. A 27-year-old woman is generally unwell and feverish with unusually dark urine. The next day, she feels much worse and has diarrhoea and vomiting, with chills and sweating. Her temperature is 38.5°C. She last visited her GP 4 months ago for travel vaccinations prior to a holiday in Kenya.

12. A 3-year-old girl has had fever and vomiting for 2 days. She is not eating, not sleeping well, and is crying more than usual. For the last day, she has been very clingy and lethargic, not showing interest in toys or games. She has a pink rash on her trunk that does not fade when pressed and she is lethargic and floppy. Her temperature is 39°C.

13. A 40-year-old man who works as a chef has had diarrhoea, vomiting, and colicky abdominal pains for 3 days. The pain is centred around his umbilicus. The diarrhoea occurs up to fives times daily and for the last day has been bloodstained. He mainly eats restaurant food, from the kitchen of the restaurant he works in.

14. A 19-year-old woman is in her first term at university. She has had a cough for the last 7 days, which is gradually getting worse. She has left-sided chest pain and is coughing up green sputum. She looks flushed, with a temperature of 39°C, a respiratory rate of 28/min, and a pulse rate of 110bpm Her chest sounds clear on auscultation.

15. A 3-year-old girl has had a high temperature since the morning. She is off her food but is still drinking. She is clingy and her stools have been loose. She is snuffly and has a rough cough, with a barking quality. Her temperature is 40°C and she is miserable but alert.

Causes of hypertension

For each patient scenario, choose the *single* most appropriate antihypertensive to prescribe from the list of options below. Each option may be used once, more than once, or not at all. ★ ★

A Atenolol

B Bendroflumethiazide

C Clonidine

D Doxazosin

E Furosemide

F Guanethidine

G Lisinopril

H Methyldopa

I Nifedipine

J No medications

K Propranolol

L Valsartan

16. A 36-year-old woman in the first trimester of pregnancy has had repeated blood pressure measurements of over 145/95mmHg before and during pregnancy, but has no evidence of proteinuria or oedema.

17. A 65-year-old man with gout has persistently raised blood pressure of 160/98mmHg and has never been on blood pressure treatment.

18. A 45-year-old man has raised blood pressure of 150/100mmHg, and is currently on no treatment.

19. A 34-year-old civil servant has a blood pressure of 135/80mmg Hg. He is currently taking citalopram for panic disorder.

20. A 50-year-old woman is currently on enalapril to control her blood pressure. Her blood pressure is now 155/90mmHg. She also has impaired glucose tolerance.

Causes of ENT problems

For each clinical situation, choose the *single* best management option from the list of options below. Each option may be used once, more than once, or not at all. ★ ★

A   Combined antibiotic and steroid ear drops

B   Nasal antihistamine spray

C   Olive oil ear drops

D   Oral aciclovir

E   Oral antibiotics

F   Oral antihistamine

G   Reassure and review within 3 weeks

H   Refer for audiometry

I   Refer to the practice nurse for ear syringing

J   Routine ENT referral

K   Saline ear drops

L   Urgent Emergency Department referral

M   Urgent ENT referral

21. A 35-year-old man has had a decline in his hearing over the last few months. He has bilateral impacted wax in his ear canals.

22. A 25-year-old swimmer has had a painful left ear for 2 days. The left ear canal is red and swollen and there is some yellow crusting. The tympanic membrane can be seen and is intact.

23. A 35-year-old woman has hurt her right ear today while cleaning it with a cotton bud. There is swelling of the ear canal and the tympanic membrane is not visible due to the swelling and the presence of blood.

24. A 4-year-old boy is brought in by his mother who thinks that his hearing is reduced. He is interacting normally with his family and is generally well.

25. A 55-year-old man has increasing pain and hearing loss in his left ear. There are crusting vesicles in the ear canal.

205

Single Best Answers

1. C ★   OHGP → p230

BMI is calculated by weight in kilograms divided by height in metres squared (kg/m²). It is a measure of weight for height and does not represent body fat or other ratios.

2. A ★   OHCS 8th edn → p770

Retention of urine and faeces should raise suspicions of cauda equina syndrome; compression of the cauda equina in the spinal canal. Pain and inability to straight leg raise can be caused in muscular back injury or sciatica, and ankle jerks are usually brisk in cord compression.

3. C ★   OHGP → pp48–49

All competent patients have a right to confidentiality and you should not break this unless the patient specifically consents for you to share the information. However, if the mother wants to give her concerns about her daughter, it is acceptable to listen to these without revealing information.

→ http://www.gmc-uk.org/guidance/current/library/confidentiality.asp

4. E ★

There are several risk factors for stroke, some of which can be modified and some of which cannot. Hypertension is considered the most important risk factor for stroke, with well-documented relationships between blood pressure and stroke occurrence. There is also good evidence that treating hypertension reduces the risk of stroke.

5. C ★   OHCS 8th edn → p532; OHGP → pp44–45

An approach that is patient-centred and identifies, acknowledges, and respects the patient's decisions and feelings ensures a better long-term result. It is important to realise that all patients have different life factors that may impact on their decision-making. Respecting these is vital in building a lasting relationship.

6. D ★

All of these are possible risk factors for poor sleep, apart from moderate cigarette smoking. However, the suggestion of low mood and possible depression is an important presenting symptom that needs to be followed up.

7. E ★

HPV types 16 and 18 can cause cervical abnormalities that may progress to become cancer. The HPV vaccine protects against these. It is currently being offered to all 12–13-year-old girls and there is a catch-up programme until 2011, which will offer the vaccine to all girls aged 13–18 years.

→ http://www.immunisation.nhs.uk/vaccines/HPV/
→ http://www.dh.gov.uk/en/Publichealth/Healthprotection/ Immunisation/Greenbook/index.htm (DoH: Immunization Against Infectious Disease – 'The Green Book')

8. D ★

9. E ★   OHCS 8th edn → p530; OHGP → p230

Type 2 diabetes is greatly increased in overweight people and is a major cause of morbidity. A healthy body mass index (BMI) is in the range of 20–25 kg/m². If this woman lost 20kg, her weight would be 65kg. Her BMI would therefore be 65/1.6², which is 25.4 kg/m², a much healthier BMI and an achievable range to aim for.

→ http://www.nice.org.uk/nicemedia/pdf/word/CG43NICEGuideline.doc

10. D ★

A possible diagnosis is malaria, which would be suspected if he had travelled to a region where malaria is prevalent.

11. D ★   OHGP → pp481, 490

Influenza vaccine is prepared each year from viruses of the three strains thought most likely to cause flu that winter. It is about 70% effective, and protection lasts for one year. Pneumococcal vaccine only needs to be given once. Both are recommended for high-risk groups of patients, including patients with diabetes.

12. E ★

Whilst all patients are entitled to appropriate treatment, you should not place other patients or practice staff at risk of harm. This patient has the right to treatment just like others, but you should not disadvantage other patients by seeing him first, simply because he is demanding. It may be necessary to call the police, but you may well be able to advise and treat him without difficulty, and you should endeavour to do this before taking more drastic action.

13. D ★   OHGP → p111

The occupational therapist's role is to assess patients in their activities of daily living and advise on how to make these achievable.

14. B ★

Glandular fever or infectious mononucleosis, caused by Epstein–Barr virus, can cause splenomegaly. A rare but serious complication is splenic rupture, the risk of which is increased by contact sports and trauma to the area. The splenomegaly usually lasts 6–8 weeks.

15. D ★   OHCS 8th edn → p301; OHGP → p750

The Pill can increase the risk of ischaemic stroke. Women who have migraine should stop the Pill immediately if they develop aura and worsening headache and should have an ischaemic event excluded if these symptoms persist. The progestogen-only pill is a safe alternative as it contains no oestrogen, which is the component that leads to the increased risk.

→ http://www.bnf.org/bnf (See section 7.3.1. Requires registration)

16. B ★

NSAIDs may cause worsening of asthma, although this is not always the case. However, the patient should be warned of the risk and advised not to take the medication. The most effective way to ensure this is done is to speak to her yourself. A further appointment can be offered to discuss alternative treatments later.

17. C ★   OHCS 8th edn → p474; OHGP → pp56–57

The health visitor is a qualified nurse with a Health Visiting qualification (includes public health nursing and health promotion). She takes over home visiting of new mothers from the midwife when the baby is 10 days old.

18. E ★   OHCS 8th edn → p384

There is a high probability that this woman has anorexia nervosa, and with a persistently low BMI below 17 kg/m², she needs to be assessed and managed by a psychiatrist with a particular interest in eating disorders. You may of course continue to see her as a GP, but she needs specialist help to direct her treatment.

19. C ★   OHCS 8th edn → p48

Pre-eclampsia is defined by hypertension plus proteinuria, plus or minus peripheral oedema. However, the presence of symptoms such as headache makes hospital referral important here. The presence of seizures would make the diagnosis eclampsia, rather than pre-eclampsia.

20. B ★

Only glomerulonephritis is an important complication of streptococcal sore throat, and it can usually be prevented by appropriate antibiotic treatment.

21. B ★★   OHGP → pp142–151

Many patients seek complementary therapies, so it is useful to have some idea of the more common ones and those for which there is an evidence base. Glucosamine may be helpful in large-joint arthritis.
→ http://jama.ama-assn.org/cgi/content/abstract/283/11/1469

22. D ★   OHGP → p119

He would qualify for free prescriptions if he was aged over 60 years, and if he had a low income and less than £16,000 in savings or investments, or if he had one of a number of chronic diseases. Help is based on a comparison between your weekly income and assessed requirements at the time the claim is made (or the date the charge was paid if a refund is claimed).
→ http://www.nhsbsa.nhs.uk/HealthCosts/Documents/HealthCosts/HC11.pdf

23. D ★★

This patient clearly has a significant urinary tract infection and needs antibiotic treatment. Trimethoprim and nalidixic acid are contraindicated in the first trimester of pregnancy, and amoxicillin, whilst safe, is likely to be ineffective due to widespread resistance. Nitrofurantoin is safe in early pregnancy but is best avoided near term because of a possible risk of haemolytic anaemia in newborn babies.

24. C ★★

Blood pressure measurement needs to be performed reliably and safely. Whilst most clinical trials in the past have used mercury sphygmomanometer readings, these are no longer considered appropriate for safety reasons. Wrist and aneroid devices are less reliable, and ambulatory readings are only appropriate for certain patients.

25. D ★★   OHCS 8th edn → p402

The patient may have capacity but it needs to be assessed. If he is competent, then he can refuse or accept any treatment offered. However, he cannot insist on treatment that is not considered appropriate by his doctor. This legal situation is covered by different Acts in England and Wales, and Scotland.

26. A ★★

Provided you are happy that a patient is not at risk of harm, it is appropriate to facilitate a referral to a complementary therapist if they request it. However, because this is a private referral, you need to ensure it is done professionally, ensuring that the patient has as much choice as possible, and that there is no suggestion that you have a personal interest in the referral.

27. C ★★

A wide variety of symptoms can occur in depression. However, it is important always to revisit the diagnosis and to assess every presentation fully. In an elderly woman with headaches and myalgia, loss of vision may occur in giant cell arteritis, and prompt treatment can save sight.

28. E ★★

Prescriptions for controlled drugs must be indelible and include:

- The name and address of the patient
- The form and strength of the preparation
- The total quantity in both words and figures of the preparation, or the number in both words and figures of dosage units, to be supplied
- The dose to be given
- The prescriber's name, signature, and address
- The date of the prescription

Pharmacists cannot dispense unless the prescription is filled in correctly.
→http://www.bnf.org/bnf/bnf/57/29424.htm (Requires registration)

29. A ★★★

When asking a patient whether they will allow a student to be present, you should have an appropriate mechanism to ensure this that does not pressurize the patient, embarrass either them or the student, or disadvantage the patient in any way.

30. A ★★★ OHCS 8ᵗʰ edn→ p144

Neonates with significant exposure to chickenpox or shingles should receive ZIG as soon as possible. The fact that the mother has probably never had chickenpox means that she has no varicella antibodies to pass across the placenta, and the baby therefore has no protection.

Extended Matching Questions

1. L ⋆

Shingles is a reactivation of latent chickenpox and the pain of shingles usually pre-dates the vesicular rash by 2–3 days. It can be confused with other conditions, as the skin looks clear in the early stages and the pain can be very severe. Shingles develops from the dorsal root ganglion it has been latent within, and therefore never crosses the midline. It also follows the line of the dermatome, sometimes also within an adjacent dermatome.

2. K ⋆

A pulmonary embolus should be suspected in anyone presenting with chest pain and shortness of breath following an operation, especially if the patient is not anticoagulated. In this case, the long-haul flight home is an additional risk factor. Other risk factors include smoking, the oral contraceptive pill, pregnancy or puerperium, malignancy, and a past history of deep vein thrombosis or pulmonary embolism. Many of the signs of pulmonary embolism are also common in patients without a pulmonary embolus, which is why the history is so important to raise suspicion of the diagnosis. This patient would need urgent referral to hospital.

3. B ⋆

Chest wall causes of pain are among the commonest reasons for chest pain seen by GPs. Sometimes the patient may describe repetitive movements or unaccustomed activity that might account for the development of the pain. Costochondritis is one of the more common presentations of musculoskeletal chest pain. It is a diffuse pain syndrome, in which multiple areas of tenderness are found that reproduce the described pain. The upper costal cartilages at the costochondral or costosternal junctions are most frequently involved.

4. F ⋆

This patient is having a myocardial infarction (MI) unless proven otherwise. It is difficult to tell the difference between acute MI and unstable angina in general practice, but the treatment is similar. An ECG may look normal at this stage. He needs urgent admission to hospital for consideration of thrombolysis or angioplasty, as this needs to be given as soon as possible. He should also be given aspirin (300mg) immediately if there is no contraindication, and he may need IV diamorphine and an anti-emetic. If his systolic blood pressure was >90mmHg and his pulse rate >100/bpm, he should also have sublingual glyceryl trinitrate to act as a coronary vasodilator.

5. H ★

Initial evaluation should consider disorders that are known to involve the pericardium, such as uraemia, recent myocardial infarction, and prior cardiac surgery. Other causes include infection (e.g. Coxsackie virus, tuberculosis), malignancy, trauma, connective tissue disease, and hypothyroidism. The examination should pay particular attention to auscultation for a pericardial friction rub and the signs associated with tamponade. The patient should be assessed that day by a cardiologist, and if it is thought to be due to an uncomplicated viral pericarditis, can be treated as an outpatient with non-steroidal anti-inflammtory drugs to control the pain and inflammation.

6. A ★

Benign positional vertigo lasts only a few seconds or minutes, and occurs with sudden changes of position. It may be caused by otoliths in the labyrinth of the inner ear, and is common after head injury or viral illness, and increases in diabetes. Diagnosis is made by history and a positive Hallpike test: sit the patient up with legs extended and rotate the head 45°; ask them to lie down quickly with the head extended; after about 10s, rotational nystagmus will occur with the fast phase towards the affected ear. The condition is self-limiting.

7. F ★

These are the symptoms and signs of hypoglycaemia. On this day, he had to start work early and had not had time to get his usual mid-morning snack, resulting in a hypoglycaemic attack. The diagnosis is made quickly on checking his capillary blood glucose.

8. L ★

Viral labyrinthitis usually follows a viral respiratory tract infection. It can be treated symptomatically with labyrinthine sedatives, such as cyclizine or prochlorperazine. It usually resolves in 2–3 weeks. If the symptoms persist for more than 6 weeks, the patient should be referred to ENT.

9. C ★

This patient is demonstrating signs of cerebellar dysfunction. The cause of this is not known from this history and examination, and the patient will need to be referred urgently for further tests including a CT brain scan. The most likely diagnosis is of a cerebellar stroke, but she could also have a cerebellar tumour or multiple sclerosis, amongst other possible diagnoses.

10. G ★

This is a complex of symptoms including clustering of attacks of vertigo and nausea, tinnitus, a sense of fullness in the ear, and sensorineural deafness, which may be progressive. All cases should be referred for confirmation of the diagnosis – in this case, the unilateral nature of her symptoms would mean an acoustic neuroma should be excluded.

General feedback on 6–10: OHCS 8ᵗʰ edn → p554–555 Dizziness is a non-specific term used by patients to describe symptoms, so getting as precise a description of the sensation as possible is vital for establishing the cause. The distribution of causes varies with age. Patients often experience vertigo as an illusion of motion; some interpret this as self-motion, others as motion of the environment. All vertigo is made worse by moving the head. This is a very useful symptom for distinguishing vertigo from other forms of dizziness. The presence of additional neurological signs strongly suggests the presence of a central vestibular lesion. Symptoms such as staggering or ataxic gait, vomiting, headache, double vision, visual loss, slurred speech, numbness of the face or body, weakness, clumsiness, or inco-ordination should be reviewed with the patient. Positional changes in symptoms, orthostatic blood pressure and pulse changes, observation of gait, and detection of nystagmus are helpful on physical examination.

11. E ★

Malaria should be excluded first, by doing a full blood count and thin and thick films to look for malaria parasites. If she is clinically very unwell, she needs urgent admission.

Malaria is a notifiable disease, 2000 cases per year are notified in the UK. *Plasmodium falciparum* malaria can be fatal in <24h, especially if it occurs in very young children.

12. F ★

A non-blanching rash with a floppy lethargic child is highly suggestive of meningococcal sepsis. The GP should call 999 and get her into hospital quickly. She or he should also give her a stat IM bolus of benzylpenicillin – for a 3-year-old child it should be 600mg (1.2g for an adult/child >10years; 300mg for infant <1year).

13. B ★

The GP should send off a stool sample for analysis. In the meantime, he or she should ask the chef not to go into work until a clear stool sample has been obtained. If the stool sample is positive for *Campylobacter*, the GP should notify Public Health and treat the patient with ciprofloxacin.

14.1 ★

The clinical findings may not show a left-sided consolidation – you may need to make the decision based on her overall clinical condition. The British Thoracic Society has guidelines for assessing the severity of community-acquired pneumonia. As this woman is tachycardic and tachypnoeic, she may need admission for IV antibiotics.

→ http://www.brit-thoracic.org.uk/Portals/0/Clinical%20Information/ Pneumonia/Guidelines/MACAPrevisedApr04.pdf

15.0 ★

She probably has a mild form of croup, which is a viral infection. She needs fluids and paracetamol, and the GP should give the parents details of symptoms they should look out for, or guidelines on when to call the doctor again if she is not getting better (for example, a non-blanching rash, if she stops drinking, or if her temperature is not controlled by paracetamol).

→ http://www.nice.org.uk/nicemedia/pdf/CG47NICEGuideline.pdf

16. H ★ ★

17. I ★ ★

18. G ★ ★

19. J ★ ★

20. I ★ ★

General feedback on 16–20: In England and Wales, the National Institute for Health and Clinical Excellence (NICE) has produced a guideline for the treatment of hypertension. This covers lifestyle factors that should be considered and modified first, and assessment of other risk factors, such as age and ethnicity. The choice of treatment (or no treatment) depends on these factors. The Scottish Intercollegiate Guidelines Network (SIGN) in Scotland has a similar guideline. Concurrent medical conditions may affect which treatment should be given; for example diuretics can be harmful in gout. In pregnancy, methyldopa is usually the drug of choice but is not used routinely elsewhere.

→ http://www.nice.org.uk/CG034
→ http://www.sign.ac.uk/guidelines/fulltext/49/section5.html
→ http://bnf.org/bnf/bnf/current/2534.htm (registration required)

21. C ★★

Olive oil drops help the ear to clean itself and are effective for excess wax causing symptoms. Syringing can lead to an increased risk of ear infections and perforations so is not a first-line treatment.

22. A ★★

This is otitis externa, infection of the external auditory meatus. Combined drops are the most effective treatment for this.

23. M ★★

Cotton buds can damage the ear, cause trauma and infection, and actually push wax further down and cause it to become impacted. In this case, there seems to be an acute injury and possibly damage to the tympanic membrane, which might need intervention.

24. H ★★

As children cannot tell you whether their hearing is reduced, parental concern should always be taken seriously. Audiometry will tell you whether he does have impaired hearing, which could be due to a number of causes, but the commonest is fluid in the middle ear.

25. D ★★

Herpes zoster (shingles) in the ear causes pain and vesicles. It can progress to hearing loss, vertigo, and facial palsy. As it is viral, it can be treated with aciclovir.

General feedback on 21–25: OHCS 8th edn → pp538, 540, 542

CHAPTER 6
ENT

Philippa Tostevin

ENT is a fascinating surgical specialty, involved in the diagnosis and management of a vast range of diseases presenting from birth through all ages. The pathologies covered range from congenital airway obstruction in the neonate to head and neck malignancies in elderly patients. Systemic diseases can also manifest for the first time in the ENT area. The creation of a surgical airway in the form of a tracheostomy can be life-saving but some ENT surgery is performed to improve quality of life, so it is particularly important to understand the indications for surgical interventions. Unlike other surgical specialties, many of the patients seen in the outpatient setting do not need surgery, and medical management is required.

For those interested in ENT surgery as a career, there are different areas within this diverse field that can be followed to a specialist level: rhinology, otology, and neuro-otology, in addition to the specialist areas of paediatric ENT, head and neck cancer surgery, voice, and facial plastic surgery.

A thorough knowledge and understanding of the diagnosis and management of common ENT conditions is vital for those wishing to work in general practice, paediatrics, or emergency medicine. ENT conditions in children provide a very large portion of the workload in any general practice setting. Various foreign bodies can be swallowed, inhaled, or inserted into the nose or ear, so an understanding of how and when these need be removed is essential for any junior doctor working in the Emergency Department.

In this chapter, the questions are based on the important knowledge that needs to be accrued as an undergraduate, as many readers may not have the opportunity to work as a junior doctor in an ENT team before treating ENT patients in the emergency department or in a general practice setting. ∎

ENT
SINGLE BEST ANSWERS

1. A 78-year-old man has sudden onset of hoarse voice. He has a weak cough and he coughs when eating. He has been a smoker since the age of 18. He has a right-sided vocal cord palsy. Which is the single most likely anatomical site for his primary malignancy? ★

A Bronchus

B Larynx

C Oesophagus

D Oral cavity

E Parotid

2. A 32-year-old lorry driver has had a painless, discharging left ear for 10 years. His Weber test lateralizes to the left and his Rinne test is negative on the left and positive on the right. The external auditory meatus is filled with mucopurulent debris. Which is the single most likely diagnosis? ★

A Chronic otitis externa

B Chronic secretory otitis media

C Chronic suppurative otitis media

D Malignant otitis externa

E Middle ear effusion

3. A 66-year-old man has a unilateral, non-pulsatile tinnitus that is keeping him awake at night. His pure tone audiogram shows asymmetrical sensorineural hearing loss. Which single benign tumour may be responsible for these findings? ★

A Astrocytoma

B Glioma

C Meningioma

D Pleomorphic adenoma

E Vestibular schwannoma

4. A 76-year-old woman has right-sided otalgia and vertigo. Her Rinne test is positive in both ears and her Weber test lateralizes to the left ear. There are vesicles present on the superior aspect of her right pinna and drooping of her face on the right side. Which single virus is most likely to have caused this clinical presentation? ★

A Adenovirus

B Cytomegalovirus

C Epstein–Barr virus

D Herpes simplex virus

E Varicella -zoster virus

5. A 23-year-old man has a 2cm ulcer in his oral cavity. He has lost 3kg in weight over the last 3 months. The edge of the ulcer is biopsied and the histopathology result shows non-caseating granulomata. Which is the single most likely diagnosis? ★

A Actinomycosis

B Crohn's disease

C Tuberculosis

D Ulcerative colitis

E Vitamin B$_{12}$ deficiency

6. A 23-year-old woman has had a fall at the gym. She now has a transient sensation of movement when she turns her head to the right. There is no hearing loss or tinnitus. Which is the single most likely diagnosis? ★

A Benign paroxysmal positional vertigo

B Labyrinthitis

C Ménière's disease

D Temporal bone fracture

E Vestibular neuronitis

7. A 17-year-old man has sudden-onset hearing loss after standing near an exploding firework. He has a central perforation of the tympanic membrane and a conductive hearing loss. Which is the single most appropriate acute management? ★

A Emergency myringoplasty

B Grommet insertion

C Intravenous antibiotics

D Keep ear dry and review

E Topical antibiotic and steroid drops

8. A 26-year-old man has had a foul smelling, painless otorrhoea and a conductive hearing loss for 3 years. There is moist white debris in the attic of the right tympanic membrane. Which is the single most appropriate next intervention? ★

A Daily suction toilet

B Intravenous antibiotics

C Mastoid exploration

D Myringoplasty

E Ventilation tube insertion

9. A 63-year-old man has otalgia and a hard, craggy mass on the right tonsil. He has been a smoker for the last 40 years. Which is the single most likely histological type of tumour? ★

A Adenocarcinoma

B Lymphoma

C Rhabdomyosarcoma

D Small cell carcinoma

E Squamous cell carcinoma

10. A 75-year-old woman has had a hoarse voice, lethargy and weight gain for 8 weeks. On examination, her vocal cords appear thickened. Which single blood test is most likely to be helpful in making a diagnosis? ★

A Full blood count

B Liver function test

C Serum calcium

D Thyroid function test

E Urea and electrolytes

11. A 3-year-old girl is snoring so loudly that she is keeping the family awake. She has never had tonsillitis, but an overnight sleep study has shown desaturations to 80% in room air when she is asleep. The oropharyngeal examination is shown in Plate 6.1. Which is the single most appropriate management? ★

A Adenotonsillectomy

B Continuous home oxygen at night

C Continuous positive airway pressure (CPAP) via a face mask at night

D Palatal stiffening procedure

E Tonsillectomy

12. A 63-year-old diabetic man has an intensely itchy and painful right ear. Spores are seen in the external auditory meatus, which are cleared with microsuction. Which is the single most appropriate management? ★

A Aluminium acetate ear drops

B Glycerine and ichthammol

C Intravenous voriconazole

D Oral ketoconazole

E Topical clotriamazole

13. A 2-year-old boy has a temperature of 39°C and purulent otorrhoea. His pinna is laterally and inferiorly displaced, but the post-auricular sulcus is maintained. Which is the single most appropriate first-line emergency management? ★

A Admit for analgesia and observation

B Admit for intravenous antibiotics

C Emergency grommet insertion

D Give antibiotic ear drops

E Give oral antibiotics

14. A 70-year-old man has had an intermittently discharging ear for 5 years. He has come for review. Which single new clinical finding would indicate that he may have developed a malignancy? ★

A Black spores in the external auditory meatus

B Circumferential oedema of the external auditory meatus

C Offensive-smelling discharge

D Purulent discharge

E Sanguinous discharge

15. A 20-year-old man has chronic facial pain and rhinorrhoea. He has had multiple courses of antibiotics with little improvement in his symptoms. A coronal CT scan of his paranasal sinuses shows a round opacity with mixed density within the right maxillary sinus. Which is the single most likely explanation for these findings? ★ ★

A Allergic polyp

B Angiofibroma

C Antrochoanal polyp

D Fungal ball

E Foreign body within the sinus

16. A 4-year-old boy with Down's syndrome has a proven middle-ear effusion bilaterally that has been present for 6 months. His pure tone hearing thresholds are 40dB bilaterally. Which is the single most appropriate management? ★ ★

A Adenoidectomy

B Bilateral mastoidectomy

C Bilateral ventilation tube insertion

D Cochlea implantation

E Watch and wait for 3 months

17. A 68-year-old woman has otalgia and dysphagia. She has angular cheilitis and pale conjunctivae. Her oropharyngeal examination is normal. In which single anatomical site is this patient likely to have a tumour? ★ ★

A Lower oesophagus

B Nasopharynx

C Post-cricoid

D Thyroid

E Tonsil

18. A 47-year-old woman has pulsatile tinnitus in her right ear. Her hearing is normal. There is a red lesion visible on the promontory in the middle ear behind the tympanic membrane. Which is the single most likely diagnosis? ★ ★

A Arteriovenous malformation

B Carotid body tumour

C Glomus tumour

D Middle-ear polyp

E Otosclerosis

19. A 72-year-old woman with rheumatoid arthritis has hoarseness of her voice. There is a left vocal cord palsy. Which single joint is likely to be involved? ★ ★

A Atlanto-occipital

B Cricoarytenoid

C Cricothyroid

D Costochondral

E Sternoclavicular

20. A 32-year-old woman is having intermittent episodes of vertigo. Each episode lasts up to 12h, with associated tinnitus and hearing loss. Which single medication may be of help in reducing the frequency of her vertiginous episodes? ★ ★

A Amitriptyline

B Betahistine

C Cyclizine

D Paroxetine

E Prochlorperazine

21. A 2-year-old girl had an episode of acute otitis media 3 weeks ago. She now has no pain or temperature, but has a residual hearing loss. A type B tympanometry trace is found with a normal canal volume measurement. Which is the single most likely explanation for this result? ★ ★

A Cholesteatoma

B Chronic suppurative otitis media

C Perforation of the tympanic membrane

D Persistent acute otitis media

E Serous middle-ear effusion

22. A 5-year-old boy has a submandibular lump. It is non-tender with a light purplish discolouration of the overlying skin. He is apyrexial and otherwise well. His GP has tried several courses of antibiotics, but it has continued to grow. Which is the single most likely diagnosis? ★ ★

A Atypical mycobacterial infection

B Brucellosis

C Infectious mononucleosis

D Lymphoma

E Toxoplasmosis

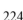

23. A 76-year-old man has acute disabling vertigo with nausea and vomiting. He has no tinnitus, and normal hearing. He has an intention tremor. Which single test would be most helpful in establishing a diagnosis? ★ ★

A Audiogram

B Brainstem-evoked response testing

C Caloric testing

D CT scan of brain

E Otoacoustic emissions

24. A 2-year-old boy was playing with a small plastic toy and then began coughing for 2min. His mother called 999. He is now completely well and eating and drinking normally but the toy is nowhere to be found. Which is the single most appropriate management? ★ ★ ★

A CT scan of the chest

B Microlaryngoscopy and bronchoscopy

C Nasendoscopy in the Emergency Department

D Flexible oesophagogastroduodenoscopy

E Rigid oesophagoscopy

25. A 23-year-old woman has fallen from a tree onto her face. She has a nasal fracture and clear rhinorrhoea. The nasal discharge is positive for glucose. Which single test would you ask for to confirm the nature of the nasal fluid? ★ ★ ★

A Albumin

B β-Galactosidase

C β-2 Transferrin

D Ferritin

E Myoglobin

26. A 16-year-old boy sustains a nasal fracture during a game of football. He feels that his nose is obstructed. Both nasal bones are in the midline and both nasal airways are obscured by red, swollen mucosa, which is soft when palpated. Which is the single most appropriate first step in management? ★ ★ ★

A Incision and drainage

B Manipulation of the nasal fracture

C Oral antibiotics and review

D Rhinoplasty

E Septoplasty

27. At 7pm, a 3-year-old girl comes to the Emergency Department having put a lithium battery up her nose earlier in the afternoon. It cannot be removed in the department. Which is the single most appropriate time to list her for removal of the battery under general anaesthetic? ★ ★ ★

A After a course of steroids to decrease the inflammation

B After waiting a few days for the inflammation to subside

C On the next available elective list

D This evening, as soon as possible

E Tomorrow morning

28. Following his laryngectomy operation, a 74-year-old man has his speech restored using a valve in a tracheo-oesophageal fistula. The speech therapist wishes to explain to him the mechanism whereby he is able to communicate again. Which is the single best description of the mechanism for his post-laryngectomy speech restoration? ★ ★ ★ ★

A A hand-held resonating device is used in conjunction with the valve to create speech

B A fenestrated tracheostomy tube is fitted to enable speech restoration

C Air from the lungs is diverted through the valve and up to the pharynx, which vibrates to create sound

D Air from the lungs is diverted through the valve, which vibrates to create sound

E Air is taken into the oesophagus and this causes the valve to vibrate

29. A 37-year-old man has an epistaxis that has not been controlled with 24h of nasal packing and bed rest. His blood pressure is 120/72mmHg. A decision for arterial ligation is made. Which single artery is most commonly ligated first in this situation? ★ ★ ★ ★

A External carotid

B Greater palatine

C Maxillary

D Posterior ethmoid

E Sphenopalatine

EXTENDED MATCHING QUESTIONS

Causes of head and neck lumps

For each of the following patients with a neck lump, choose the *single* most likely diagnosis from the list below. Each answer can be used once, more than once, or not at all. ★

A Anaplastic carcinoma

B Branchial cyst

C Carotid body tumour

D Dermoid cyst

E Graves' disease

F Hashimoto's thyroiditis

G Lipoma

H Lymphoma

I Multinodular goitre

J Papillary thyroid cancer

K Sebaceous cyst

L Thyroglossal cyst

M Toxoplasmosis

1. A 40-year-old man has multiple soft lymph nodes in the posterior triangle. He has lost weight and has had night sweats for the last 6 weeks.

2. A 15-year-old girl has a painless, midline lump that transilluminates and moves with protrusion of the tongue.

3. An 18-year-old man has a painless lump anterior to the upper third of the sternomastoid on the left. It is under the skin and is soft, fluctuant, and non-tender.

4. A 74-year-old woman has a hard irregular midline lump, difficulty swallowing, and stridor.

5. A 40-year-old woman has a smooth midline lump that moves with swallowing. She has protruberant eyes and a tremor of her hands.

Securing the airway

For each emergency airway scenario, choose the *single* most appropriate initial step to secure the airway from the list of options below. Each option may be used once, more than once, or not at all. ★

A Cricothyroidotomy

B Endotracheal intubation

C Laryngeal mask airway

D Nasal cannulae

E Nasopharyngeal airway

F Nebulized aceylcysteine

G Nebulized adrenaline (epinephrine)

H Nebulized ipratropium

I Nebulized salbutamol

J Oral chlorphenamine

K Oral prednisolone

L Oropharyngeal airway

M Tracheostomy

6. A 66-year-old woman is extubated following an elective thyroidectomy. She is still quite sleepy and has no gag reflex. Her airway needs protection to take her to the recovery room.

7. A 30-year-old man is having a picnic. He suddenly chokes on his sandwich. His friend attempts the Heimlich manoeuvre but is unsuccessful. When the paramedics arrive, he is deeply cyanosed and loses consciousness.

8. A 3-year-old boy is in respiratory distress with inspiratory stridor, drooling, and tracheal tug.

9. A 25-year-old man is involved in a motor vehicle collision and sustains bilateral maxillary and mandibular fractures. His airway needs protection whilst his facial fractures heal.

10. A 14-year-old girl is acutely short of breath following a school sports day. She has widespread expiratory wheeze throughout both lung fields.

Causes of nasal obstruction

For each patient, choose the *single* most likely cause of
nasal obstruction from the list of options below. Each
option may be used once, more than once, or not at all. ★

A Adenoiditis

B Allergic rhinitis

C Aspergilloma

D Atrophic rhinitis

E Candidiasis

F Maxillary sinusitis

G Mucormycosis

H Nasal polyps

I Osteomyelitis

J Rhinitis medicamentosa

K Sarcoidosis

L Tuberculosis

M Vasomotor rhinitis

11. A 56-year-old man who is a wine taster is unable to work due to anosmia. He also has uncontrollable, bilateral, watery rhinorrhoea and mild asthma.

12. A 3-year-old boy has bilateral mucopurulent rhinorrhoea and halitosis. He is mouth breathing and also has a conductive hearing loss.

13. A 27-year-old man has unilateral purulent rhinorrhoea and left-sided facial pain following a dental extraction.

14. A 23-year-old woman has had a left-sided frontal headache and bilateral purulent rhinorrhoea for 4 weeks. She has a soft mass overlying the left frontal sinus.

15. A 20-year-old man has a cough and severe, red, indurated nasal crusting requiring debridement. He also has peripheral oedema, with swollen, painful fingers.

Causes of facial palsy

For each of the following patients with facial palsy, choose the *single* most likely diagnosis from the list below. Each answer can be used once, more than once, or not at all. ★

A Acute otitis media

B Adenocarcinoma of the parotid

C Cerebral oedema

D Cholesteatoma

E Embolic stroke

F Haemorrhagic stroke

G Herpes simplex virus infection

H Occipital fracture

I Pleomorphic adenoma

J Sarcoidosis

K Secretory otitis media

L Temporal bone fracture

M Varicella zoster virus infection

16. A 10-year-old boy has had pain in the right ear and difficulty hearing for 2 days. He has a temperature of 38.3°C. He now has a right lower motor neurone facial palsy.

17. A 75-year-old man has a hard mass in front of his right tragus and a right lower motor neurone facial palsy.

18. A 35-year-old man has had a road traffic accident. He has a bruise over the mastoid area and a right-sided lower motor neurone facial nerve palsy.

19. A 78-year-old woman has vertigo and difficulty hearing with a right lower motor neurone facial palsy. There are small vesicles in her ear.

20. A 37-year-old man has had painless, offensive discharge from his left ear for 10 years. He has difficulty hearing and a lower motor neurone palsy on the left.

Causes of stridor

For each of the following patients with stridor, choose the *single* most likely diagnosis from the list below. Each answer can be used once, more than once, or not at all. ★

A Bilateral vocal cord palsy

B Bronchogenic carcinoma

C Diphtheria

D Infectious mononucleosis

E Laryngeal cleft

F Laryngeal haemangioma

G Laryngeal papilloma

H Laryngomalacia

I Laryngotracheobronchitis (croup)

J Leukoplakia

K Subglottic stenosis

L Supraglottitis

M Vocal cord nodules

21. A 2-week-old boy has stridor that is worse when he is lying on his back. He is pink in air and is thriving and breastfeeding well.

22. A 75-year-old man has a sudden onset of hoarseness. He has smoked 30 cigarettes a day for 40 years. On examination of the larynx, he has a left-sided vocal cord palsy.

23. A 6-year-old boy has had progressive stridor and voice change for the last 2 months. He is otherwise well and has no temperature.

24. A 70-year-old man is unwell, has difficulty swallowing, and is drooling saliva. He has a temperature of 39°C and a heart rate of 110bpm.

25. A 2-year-old boy has had a cold for 2 days. He now has a barking cough and hoarse voice and has had stridor for 24h. He has had two previous similar episodes.

Causes of thyroid pathology

For each clinical scenario, choose the *single* most likely thyroid pathology from the list of options below. Each option may be used once, more than once, or not at all. ★

A Adenoma

B Anaplastic carcinoma

C Follicular carcinoma

D Graves' disease

E Hashimoto's thyroiditis

F Lymphoma

G Medullary carcinoma

H Multinodular goitre

I Papillary carcinoma

J Pyramidal lobe cyst

K Parathyroid adenoma

L Thyroid cyst

M Toxic adenoma

26. A 66-year-old woman has weight loss and palpitations. She has a 2cm lump in the left lobe of the thyroid and the rest of the gland is impalpable. There is no palpable cervical lymphadenopathy. Her pulse rate is 100bpm and it is irregularly irregular.

27. An 84-year-old woman has a rapidly growing, irregular, hard mass in the anterior triangle of her neck. She also has dysphagia and inspiratory stridor.

28. A 24-year-old woman has a 2cm lump in the left anterior triangle at the level of the left lobe of the thyroid gland. The skin overlying the lump is normal and the lump itself is brilliantly transilluminable.

29. A 35-year-old man comes to the Emergency Department with a wrist fracture, after performing a handstand. He has a palpable mass in the left anterior triangle.

30. A 60-year-old woman has fatigue, constipation, and depression. She has diffuse enlargement of the thyroid gland.

ENT
ANSWERS

Single Best Answers

1. B ★

About a third of recurrent laryngeal nerve palsies are caused by cancers; 40% of these are in the larynx. The risk is increased in smokers. The left recurrent laryngeal nerve has a long course and loops down under the arch of the aorta in the chest, so may be affected in malignant tumours of the mediastinum. This is less common on the right. Oesophageal cancers can have pressure effects, but dysphagia would be more prominent.

2. C ★   OHCS 8th edn → p540

There is a long history of suppuration here. Chronic suppurative otitis media causes a conductive hearing loss, demonstrated by the tuning fork tests, whereas otitis externa does not.

3. E ★   OHCS 8th edn → p570

A schwannoma, or acoustic neuroma, is a slow-growing benign tumour that causes problems by local pressure on the cochlear nerve, resulting in tinnitus and hearing loss. The main differential is a meningioma, but, in this location, vestibular schwannomas are more common. However, imaging is needed to distinguish them.

4. E ★   OHCS 8th edn → p652

This is Ramsay Hunt syndrome, caused by varicella-zoster virus reactivation in a patient that has had chickenpox in the past. The combination of otalgia, hearing impaiment, vertigo, a lower motor neurone facial nerve palsy, and visible vesicles gives the diagnosis.

5. B ★

Crohn's disease causes non-caseating granulomata in the gastrointestinal (GI) tract, anywhere from the mouth to the anus, so should always be a differential diagnosis in any patient with unusual or persistent mouth ulceration, especially when coupled with other GI signs or symptoms. Tuberculosis causes caseating granulomata. Ulcerative colitis affects the colon only, not the upper GI tract.

6. A ★   OHCS 8ᵗʰ edn → pp554–555

Benign positional vertigo is common after a head injury. Attacks are provoked by head movement. Labyrinthitis usually follows a viral illness. Ménière's disease has associated tinnitus. Temporal bone fracture causes severe dizziness, often associated with facial nerve palsy and hearing loss.

7. D ★

Perforations may heal on their own, but while the drum is perforated, there is increased risk of ear infection so it is best to keep water out. Sudden loud noises often cause the most severe perforations and treatment may be needed, later such as myringoplasty.

8. C ★   OHCS 8ᵗʰ edn → p544

This man has a cholesteatoma – an area of skin in the middle ear that is locally destructive. It can be secondary to a tear in the tympanic membrane and skin grows through. If a patient has chronic discharge, this should be considered. On examination, a cottage-cheese-like discharge is seen. If left, it can invade intracranially, so surgical treatment is needed to remove the sac. A mastoidectomy may be needed.

9. E ★   OHCS 8ᵗʰ edn → p570

85% of pharyngeal cancers are squamous. Risk factors are smoking or chewing tobacco and age, and human papillomavirus infection is also an increasingly common cause.

10. D ★   OHCS 8ᵗʰ edn → p568

Hypothyroidism can cause oedema of the vocal cords and therefore hoarseness. The history of lethargy and weight gain adds further clues. The other way in which thyroid dysfunction can cause hoarseness is by pressure from a goitre. The list of causes of hoarseness is long and therefore you need to look for other clues in the history and examination.

11. A ★

Although many fewer adenotonsillectomies are performed in children these days due to the surgical morbidity, airway obstruction by tonsillar hypertrophy is an indication. This child's saturations are dipping to 80% during sleep, which indicates significant obstruction. Adenoid and tonsil tissue can be large in young children and both need to be removed. Although a Cochrane review has highlighted that there is no good-quality trial data on efficacy, this is still the most common treatment when obstruction is suspected. If this fails and there are other problems, such as significant obesity or neuromuscular problems, oxygen and CPAP may become necessary, but they are not first line. Similarly, palatal stiffening procedures, such as the insertion of implants, may be used in adults but are not appropriate in growing children.

→ http://www.cochrane.org/reviews/en/ab003136.html

12. E ★

Spores indicate a fungal infection, so an antifungal is needed. People who are immunocompromised are at increased risk of this. However, oral and IV treatments are usually not necessary as a first-line treatment, and topical treatment should be given in healthy patients. Aluminium acetate can be used as an astringent for otitis externa, but antifungals would be better in this proven fungal case.

13. B ★   OHCS 8ᵗʰ edn → p544

The high fever, thick purulent discharge, and distorted ear point to mastoiditis. The ear is typically displaced laterally and inferiorly, and there may be swelling seen over the mastoid process behind the ear. This is a serious infection and the child should be admitted and given IV antibiotics while surgical treatment is considered. Depending on the degree of damage, different surgical procedures are used to drain the pus.

14. E ★

Bloody discharge indicates a squamous cell carcinoma. This can form polyps that bleed easily on contact.

15. D ★★   OHCS 8ᵗʰ edn → p558

In any patient with chronic, recurrent sinus problems, unusual infections or causes need to be considered. An overgrowth of fungi, usually *Aspergillus* species, can form a ball in the sinuses, usually the maxillary sinus. This will look like a mass filling the sinus on scanning. Polyps look like polypoid growths coming from the lining of the sinus on a CT scan. Allergic polyps commonly occur in the ethmoid sinuses. Angiofibromas are rare and usually cause some distortion of the sinus on a CT scan; they often cause bleeding. Foreign bodies in the sinuses are rare; they sometimes happen with facial trauma.

16. C ★★   OHCS 8ᵗʰ edn → p546

Ventilation tubes, or grommets, are the treatment in glue ear, which is more common in Down's syndrome. Glue ear refers to otitis media with effusion and is the main cause of hearing loss in young children. This boy has evidence of hearing impairment on his audiograms. If left, this may seriously affect his learning and development.

17. C ★★ OHCS 8th edn → pp570–571

Post-cricoid tumours in the hypopharynx often cause the sensation of a lump in the throat before interfering with swallowing. As they grow, they cause local pain. They can also cause referred pain to the ear along the sensory fibres of the vagus nerve. This is an ominous sign. Clinical anaemia also indicates that the tumour is advanced.

18. C ★★ OHCS 8th edn → p552

A glomus tumour, or non-chromaffin paraganglionoma, is a rare vascular benign tumour that comes from the glomus body, a small collection of paraganglionic tissue. These tumours often occur in the middle ear. Because of blood flow, the tinnitus is pulsatile. A mass may also be felt in the ear. They can also occur in the carotid body, but would not give these symptoms.

19. B ★★ OHCS 8th edn → p568

The cricoarytenoid joints rotate with the vocal cords, so arthritis here causing stiffness can affect the pitch and tone of the voice. This has been reported in 17–70% of patients with rheumatoid arthritis, and airway obstruction by swelling is a rare but serious complication.

20. B ★★ OHCS 8th edn → p554

This is a description of Ménière's disease – attacks of disabling vertigo with unilateral tinnitus and progressive sensorineural deafness. Treatment is symptomatic initially. Anti-emetics such as cyclizine or prochlorperazine may help with symptoms but will not reduce the frequency of attacks. Betahistine may help, although trial results are equivocal. However, a trial is often given.

21. E ★★ OHCS 8th edn → pp540, 546

Fluid in the middle ear causes dampening of the tympanic membrane movement and results in hearing impairment and a flat trace on tympanometry. Serous effusion can occur during the resolution of an acute otitis media, probably due to Eustachian tube dysfunction. It will usually resolve by 3 months. Recurrent infections can lead to a cycle of inflammation and can cause chronic suppurative otitis media.

22. A ★★ OHCS 8th edn → p576

The characteristic appearance of this infection is an enlarging, non-tender, violaceous mass. It does not disappear following antibiotic use. It is rare, but should be considered.

23. D ★★ OHCS 8th edn → p554

The unusual feature here is the intention tremor, which should lead you to suspect a brain lesion. Vertigo caused by central lesions is rare, but features in the history may lead you to suspect these. The other tests here test hearing or assess each labyrinth in turn.

24. B ★★★

Children often choke on small foreign bodies, which may become lodged in the airway. If left, they can erode, obstruct, or cause infection and collapse. Larger objects tend to get stuck in the larynx and may cause airway obstruction or hoarseness. The majority get stuck in the bronchus and cause unilateral wheeze and breath sounds and may cause cough. Without the classic history, these may be missed or mistaken for asthma. Although inspiratory and expiratory chest X-rays may help, very young children cannot co-operate with these and a single chest film may miss the diagnosis. To look for the foreign body, you need to look carefully at the upper and lower airway by bronchoscopy.

25. C ★★★ OHCS 8th edn → p560

Clear fluid positive for glucose on a dipstick test suggests a basal skull fracture and leakage of cerebrospinal fluid (CSF). β-2 Transferrin is a protein found only in CSF and perilymph so can be used to confirm CSF rhinorrhea in suspected basal skull fracture.

26. A ★★★ OHCS 8th edn → p560

This boy has a septal haematoma, which is causing the obstruction. It is rare but serious, and, if left, can cause septal necrosis and collapse. The treatment is to drain it under general anaesthesia and pack the nose. Septoplasty or rhinoplasty may be needed later after fractures if the nose sets abnormally and causes deviation of the septum and blockage or deformity.

27. D ★★★ OHCS 8th edn → p560

Batteries are corrosive and need urgent removal.

28. C ★★★★

→ http://www.cancerhelp.org.uk/help/default.asp?page=5647

29. E ★★★★ OHCS 8th edn → p563

Ongoing epistaxis despite nasal packing is an emergency and the nose needs to be examined under anaesthesia. The sphenopalatine artery is a branch of the external carotid and passes through the sphenopalatine foramen into the back of the nose. It is distal, so ligation usually controls bleeding with few complications. Older techniques ligating the external carotid or maxillary artery have higher complication rates.

Extended Matching Questions

1. H ★

Weight loss, night sweats, and fever are worrying symptoms to specifically ask about in any patient with a neck swelling. They are known as the B symptoms in lymphoma.

2. L ★

This is the classic description of a thyroglossal cyst, a cystic swelling that develops along the thryoglossal duct.

3. B ★

This is a congenital remnant of embryonic development, resulting from failure of obliteration of the second branchial cleft. These cysts may go unnoticed for some time. The position is typical, between the sternomastoid and the pharynx, and it appears to be fluid-filled.

4. A ★

This is an aggressive form of malignancy that gives a hard, tethered goitre, often with surrounding lymphadenopathy, and presses on surrounding structures.

5. E ★

Graves' disease is an autoimmune thyroiditis. Autoantibodies stimulate thyroid-stimulating hormone receptors and cause increased thyroid hormone production. They also cause a diffuse goitre and inflammation in the eyes leading to exophthalmos. The resulting thyrotoxicosis causes symptoms and signs, including tremor.

General feedback on 1–5: OHCS 8th edn →p570

6. L ★

The oropharyngeal (Guedel) airway is suitable in patients with no gag reflex. It is easy to insert and remove.

7. A ★

In confirmed airway obstruction at or above the level of the larynx, cricothyroidotomy is the final step to provide a temporary emergency airway. It can be performed relatively quickly by emergency staff.

8. G ★

In laryngotracheobronchitis in children, nebulized steroid or adrenaline can be used to decrease laryngeal swelling. Oral dexamethasone can also be used, but prednisolone is not appropriate.

9. M ★

With significant facial injuries, airway obstruction can occur because of the swelling, so medium-term ventilation may be needed. A tracheostomy may be better than endotracheal intubation in this case.
→ http://www.sicsebm.org.uk/PercTrach/Bouderka .2004.htm

10. I ★

For wheeze, the treatment is salbutamol, which is a bronchodilatator.

General feedback on 6–10: OHCS 8th edn →p566

11. H ★

These cause a watery nasal discharge and post-nasal drip. Changes in smell are frequent.

12. A ★

Enlarged adenoids are common in children and can lead to mouth breathing, snoring, and bad breath due to airway obstruction. As they block the Eustachian tubes, they can cause dysfunction and fluid in the middle ear.

13. F ★

Dental root infection can spread to the sinuses and cause a foul discharge and cheek pain.

14. I ★

This is uncommon, but the prolonged history of purulent discharge suggests bacterial infection. The mass would be uncommon in simple sinusitis. This is also called a Pott's puffy tumour.

15. K ★

Sarcoid skin plaques often appear on the face. The collection of unusual signs and symptoms here should point towards a systemic disorder. Tuberculosis can cause cough, but would not cause the same plaque-like rash and finger swelling.

General feedback on 11–15: OHCS 8th edn →pp556, 561

16. A ★

Infection in the middle ear can spread to the facial nerve. Acute otitis media is common in children, although this complication is unusual.

17. B ★

The parotid gland lies in front of the tragus and curves around the angle of the mandible. Malignant tumours are rare (80% of masses are

pleiomorphic adenomas) but the hard texture and invasion to cause a
VIIth nerve palsy suggest this.

18. L ★

The trauma here suggests a fracture. Around 50% of transverse
temporal bone fractures will result in some facial paralysis.

19. M ★

Varicella zoster virus can infect cranial nerves VII and VIII, causing
facial paralysis, ear pain, vertigo, and hearing loss.

20. D ★

This is a serious condition, caused by skin in the middle ear and
mastoid that is locally destructive. The discharge may be ignored and
patients often present late with headache, pain, facial paralysis, and
vertigo as the cholesteatoma erodes. Treatment is surgical.

General feedback on 16–20: OHCS 8th edn → pp542–544, 570, 578

21. H ★

This is the commonest cause of stridor in neonates. Babies are usually
well and feed fine, but the stridor can be very loud and cause alarm.
It is caused by shortened aryepiglottic folds and immature, floppy
cartilage, which cause the larynx to collapse on inspiration.

22. B ★

Lung cancer can cause a recurrent laryngeal nerve palsy. The nerve
descends into the chest before passing back up to innervate the
intrinsic muscles of the larynx.

23. G ★

The chronic, progressive nature suggests that this is not acute
infection, which would be the commonest cause in children. Laryngeal
papillomas are similar to warts on the larynx, caused by human
papilloma virus, and they usually occur in children.

24. L ★

This acute history in a toxic patient suggests infection. Supraglottitis
is uncommon but is life-threatening. The inability to swallow – even
saliva – suggests airway obstruction.

25. I ★

Croup, or viral laryngotracheobronchitis, is a common illness in
children under the age of about 7 years. It is usually preceded by a
cold and progresses to a typical barking cough and stridor. It can be
recurrent.

26. M ★

A thyroid adenoma is a benign, solitary tumour. It can be silent but may produce thyroxine and cause symptoms of hyperthyroidism. In contrast, a multinodular goitre gives a diffusely lumpy gland.

27. B ★

This is an aggressive form of malignancy that gives a hard, tethered goitre, often with surrounding lymphadenopathy, and presses on surrounding structures.

28. L ★

A cyst is a fluid-filled lump, so will transilluminate.

29. K ★

A parathyroid adenoma will produce parathyroid hormone, which causes calcium resorption from bones by indirectly stimulating osteoclasts. It can therefore present with fractures caused by minimal trauma.

30. E ★

These are symptoms of hypothyroidism. Hashimoto's thyroiditis is an autoimmune disease and is the commonest cause of hypothyroidism. The gland swells as a result of being diffusely invaded by inflammatory cells.

CHAPTER 7

DERMATOLOGY

Virginia Hubbard

Skin diseases have a serious impact on an individual's quality of life. It is well recognized that conditions such as psoriasis may have a similar impact on a patient's quality of life to chronic diseases such as diabetes, hypertension, and depression.

Skin problems account for approximately 20% of all patient consultations in primary care in the UK. It is important that clinicians are able to diagnose common skin diseases such as acne, eczema, psoriasis, and cutaneous malignancies, and initiate an appropriate management plan. This requires the ability to take a full history and conduct a complete examination. A complete dermatological examination involves examination of the entire skin, mucous membranes, hair, and nails. The description of cutaneous pathologies should include the location and distribution of lesions. The morphology of a lesion or each component of a generalized eruption should be noted. Other organ systems may also need to be examined.

The questions in this chapter will test your knowledge of the skin problems frequently encountered in non-specialist clinical practice. Other more rare skin disorders are also covered, either because they are potentially life-threatening or are a sign of systemic disease. The questions are designed to improve your ability to recognize the morphology and distribution of cutaneous physical signs.

Hopefully, you will find these questions stimulating and an aid to improving your knowledge of skin disease. ■

DERMATOLOGY
SINGLE BEST ANSWERS

1. A 42-year-old man with type 2 diabetes has hyperpigmented skin in his axillae, as shown in Plate 7.1. Which is the single most likely diagnosis? ★

A Acanthosis nigricans

B Atopic eczema

C Erythrasma

D Seborrhoeic dermatitis

E Tinea corporis

2. A 28-year-old man has had red scaly patches over his cheeks for 2 years, as shown in Plate 7.2. He also has scaling of the skin around his eyebrows. Which is the single most likely diagnosis? ★

A Atopic eczema

B Candidiasis

C Psoriasis

D Seborrhoeic dermatitis

E Tinea faceii

3. A 14-year-old girl has lesions on her fingers which have been present for 5 months. They are shown in Plate 7.3. Which is the single most likely causative organism? ★

A Adenovirus

B Coxsackievirus

C Herpes simplex virus

D Human papillomavirus

E Molluscum contagiosum virus

4. A 23-year-old woman has a rash affecting her forehead, cheeks, and chin, as shown in Plate 7.4. Which is the single predominant lesion shown here? ★

A Comedone

B Macule

C Nodule

D Papule

E Pustule

5. A 30-year-old woman has had itchy skin for most of her life. Her face is shown in Plate 7.5. Which is the single most likely diagnosis? ★

A Acne rosacea

B Atopic eczema

C Impetigo

D Psoriasis

E Seborrhoeic dermatitis

6. A 38-year-old woman with lifelong atopic eczema has noticed her eczema getting worse over the past 7 days. She has been taking flucloxacillin for 4 days, but her condition is getting worse and painful, as shown in Plate 7.6. Which single treatment should be given? ★

A Betamethasone valerate ointment

B Emulsifying ointment

C IV aciclovir

D IV benzylpenicillin

E Oral metronidazole

7. A 36-year-old man has had a skin rash for 20 years, as shown in Plate 7.7. Which is the single most likely diagnosis? ★

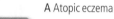

A Atopic eczema

B Lichen planus

C Pityriasis versicolor

D Psoriasis

E Seborrhoeic dermatitis

8. A 40-year-old woman attends her GP surgery for a well-woman check-up. She has multiple skin lesions, as shown in Plate 7.8, that have been present since she was a child and are slowly increasing in number. Which is the single most likely diagnosis? ★

A Epidermoid cysts

B Ganglions

C Neurofibromatosis

D Tuberous sclerosis

E Viral warts

9. A 56-year-old man has a thumb as shown in Plate 7.9. He jammed the thumb in a door a few months ago. The rest of his skin examination is normal. Which is the single most likely diagnosis? ★

A Haematoma

B Lichen planus

C Malignant melanoma

D Onychomycosis

E Psoriasis

10. A 37-year-old woman has painful, swollen, distal interpharyngeal joints. She has the nail changes shown in Plate 7.10. She says that her nails have been like this for 10 years. Which is the single most likely diagnosis? ★

A Atopic eczema

B Lichen planus

C Psoriasis

D Systemic lupus erythematosus

E Tinea manuum

11. A 40-year-old woman has had a swollen leg for 6 days, as shown in Plate 7.11. Her temperature is 38.6°C and her full blood count shows a neutrophil count of 11×10^9/L. Which is the single most likely diagnosis? ★

A Cellulitis

B Deep vein thrombosis

C Psoriasis

D Tinea corporis

E Venous eczema

12. A 40-year-old man has skin between his toes, as shown in Plate 7.12. Which is the single most likely diagnosis? ★

A Atopic eczema

B Candidiasis

C Psoriasis

D Tinea pedis

E Viral wart

13. A 5-year-old girl has had blisters on her left thigh, as shown in Plate 7.13, for 2 days. It started with a yellow crusted area 5 days ago, which spread, and then the blisters followed. She is otherwise well. Which is the single most likely diagnosis? ★

A Bullous impetigo

B Bullous pemphigoid

C Chronic bullous disease of childhood

D Insect bites

E Scabies

14. A 35-year-old woman has had a skin problem for a number of years. She had a caesarean section last year and her scar is shown in Plate 7.14. Which is the single best description of the appearance? ★

A Auspitz sign

B Impetiginization

C Keloid scar

D Köbner phenomenon

E Striae

15. A 34-year-old man has a lesion on his leg, shown in Plate 7.15. He first noticed it about 2 months ago. Which is the single most likely diagnosis? ★

A Actinic keratosis

B Benign naevus

C Bowen's disease

D Malignant melanoma

E Seborrhoeic keratosis

16. A 10-month-old baby has had skin lesions for 2 days, as shown in Plate 7.16. He had an upper respiratory tract infection last week, but seems well in himself now. The lesions seem to be in a different place from the ones he had yesterday Which is the single most likely diagnosis? ★

A Acute urticaria

B Atopic eczema

C Erythema multiforme

D Meningococcal septicaemia

E Urticaria pigmentosa

17. A 28-year-old woman developed a rash on her body 1 week ago. Today, it has spread to her hands, as shown in Plate 7.17. Three weeks ago she had a 3-day course of trimethoprim to treat a urinary tract infection. Which is the single most likely diagnosis? ★

A Acute urticaria

B Allergic contact eczema

C Erythema multiforme

D Erythema nodosum

E Psoriasis

18. A 64-year-old man has had a sore back and mouth for 2 months. These are shown in Plate 7.18(a, b). Which is the single most likely diagnosis? ★

A Bullous pemphigoid

B Erythema multiforme

C Herpes simplex virus infection

D Lichen planus

E Pemphigus vulgaris

19. A 30-year-old man with ulcerative colitis has lesions on his anterior shins. They started 7 months ago and are getting bigger. They are shown in Plate 7.19. Which is the single most likely diagnosis? ★

A Erythema nodosum

B Leucocytoclastic vasculitis

C Necrobiosis lipoidica

D Pyoderma gangrenosum

E Venous ulcers

20. A 60-year-old man has a lesion on his arm that has grown rapidly over the past 3 weeks. It is not painful. It is shown in Plate 7.20. Which is the single most likely diagnosis? ★

A Actinic keratosis

B Basal cell carcinoma

C Keratoacanthoma

D Malignant melanoma

E Seborrhoeic keratosis

21. A 22-year-old man has a lesion on his lower abdomen that is increasing in size, shown in Plate 7.21. He has tried 1% hydrocortisone cream to no avail. Which is the single most appropriate treatment? ★

A Betamethasone valerate cream

B Ketoconazole shampoo

C Oral flucloxacillin

D Oral prednisolone

E Oral terbinafine

Dermatology

22. A 45-year-old man had a cardiac transplant 8 years ago. He has developed a painful lesion on his forehead that is irregular in shape with a thick crust and has grown rapidly over the past 3 months. Which is the single most likely diagnosis? ★

A Actinic keratosis

B Bowen's disease

C Malignant melanoma

D Seborrhoeic keratosis

E Squamous cell carcinoma

23. An 18-year-old man has severe, scarring acne with multiple nodules and cysts on his face, which has been getting progressively worse over the past 5 years. Treatment with oxytetracycline for 8 months has not helped. He is otherwise well. Which is the single most appropriate treatment? ★

A 5% Benzoyl peroxide cream

B Clobetasone butyrate cream

C Oral erythromycin

D Oral isotretinoin

E Oral prednisolone

24. A 3-month-old baby has a rash in his groin. He is otherwise well. The rash is shown in Plate 7.22. Which is the single most appropriate treatment to prescribe? ★

A 1% Hydrocortisone cream

B Aqueous cream

C Fucidin cream

D No treatment

E Nystatin cream

25. A 56-year-old woman has a sore, red, dry, itchy rash confined to her face that has developed over the past month. The rest of her skin is normal. She is well and takes no medication. Which is the single most likely diagnosis? ★

A Acne rosacea

B Allergic contact dermatitis

C Atopic eczema

D Seborrhoeic dermatitis

E Systemic lupus erythematosus

26. A 69-year-old man has the appearance of his nose shown in Plate 7.23. This has been present for 9 years. Which is the single best term to describe the appearance? ★ ★

A Acne vulgaris

B Lupus pernio

C Lupus vulgaris

D Rhinophyma

E Wegener's granulomatosis

27. A 26-year-old man with atopic eczema has very itchy lesions on his palms, as shown in Plate 7.24. They come and go and seem to flare up when the rest of his eczema is bad. He has not yet tried any treatments as he is unsure what to use. Which is the single most appropriate treatment? ★ ★

A 1% Hydrocortisone ointment

B 5% Permethrin cream

C Aciclovir cream

D Betamethasone valerate ointment

E Ketoconazole cream

28. A 12-year-old boy has had atopic eczema for many years. He is concerned about paler patches on his face, as shown in Plate 7.25, which have been present for the past 6 months. He has changes consistent with eczema over the rest of his skin, but no pigmentary change. Which is the single most likely diagnosis? ★ ★

A Cutaneous T-cell lymphoma

B Pityriasis alba

C Seborrhoeic dermatitis

D Tinea facei

E Vitiligo

29. A 78-year-old woman has an itchy rash over her trunk and limbs, shown in Plate 7.26. She has been itchy for several weeks and blisters appeared last week. She takes no regular medication. Which is the single most likely diagnosis? ★ ★

A Bullous pemphigoid

B Erythema multiforme

C Pemphigus vulgaris

D Psoriasis

E Scabies

30. A 47-year-old man has had a rash over both lower legs for 2 days, as shown in Plate 7.27. He was treated with amoxicillin for a throat infection last week. Which is the single most likely diagnosis? ★ ★

A Cellulitis

B Erythema multiforme

C Erythema nodosum

D Leukocytoclastic vasculitis

E Streptococcal septicaemia

31. A 36-year-old woman is concerned about the pigmentation on her cheeks, shown in Plate 7.28, which is spreading. She takes no medication. Which is the single most appropriate treatment? ★ ★

A Betamethasone valerate cream

B High-factor sunblock

C Hydroquinone cream

D Hydroxychloroquine

E Oral prednisolone for 6 weeks

32. A 30-year-old woman gave birth 7 weeks ago. She has had a lesion on her breast for 2 weeks. It bleeds profusely and interferes with breastfeeding of her baby. Which is the single most likely diagnosis? ★ ★

A Bacillary angiomatosis

B Granuloma annulare

C Pyoderma gangrenosum

D Pyogenic granuloma

E Viral wart

33. A 30-year-old man has been on a walking holiday in Spain and now has blisters, shown in Plate 7.29. The remainder of his skin is normal. Which is the single most likely diagnosis? ★ ★

A Allergic contact eczema

B Bullous pemphigoid

C Impetigo

D Insect bite reaction

E Linear IgA disease

EXTENDED MATCHING QUESTIONS

Causes of skin lumps

For each patient with a skin lesion, choose the *single* most likely diagnosis from the list of options below. Each option may be used once, more than once, or not at all. ★

A Basal cell carcinoma

B Becker's naevus

C Benign intradermal naevus

D Dermatofibroma

E Malignant melanoma

F Pilomatricoma

G Seborrhoeic keratosis

H Squamous cell carcinoma

1. A 74-year-old woman has a lesion on her nose. It has been present for 6 months. It bleeds and crusts but never clears. It is shown in Plate 7.30.

2. A 47-year-old woman noticed a lesion on her abdomen 3 months ago. It is itchy. It has not changed in appearance. It is shown in Plate 7.31.

3. A 30-year-old woman noticed a lesion on her calf shortly after returning from holiday in Cyprus. It is shown in Plate 7.32.

4. A 35-year-old man has a lesion on his back. It was noticed by his wife. His wife has been asking him to show it to a doctor, because it has been increasing in size over the past 2 months. It is shown in Plate 7.33.

5. A 14-year-old boy has a lesion on his shoulder. It appeared at puberty. It causes him embarrassment when changing for sport. It is shown in Plate 7.34.

Causes of infections in the skin

For each patient with a rash, choose the *single* most likely causative organism from the list of options below. Each option may be used once, more than once, or not at all. ★

A *Borrelia burgdorferi*

B *Clostridium botulinum*

C *Escherichia coli*

D Herpes simplex virus

E Molluscum contagiosum virus

F *Sarcoptes scabiei*

G *Staphylococcus aureus*

H Varicella zoster virus

6. A 32-year-old woman with type 1 diabetes has a hot, red, painful leg, shown in Plate 7.35.

7. An 8-year-old girl has developed lesions around her mouth over the past 4 days, which are shown in Plate 7.36.

8. A 5-year-old boy has lesions on his abdomen that have been present for about a month. His father reports that he is developing new ones. They are shown in Plate 7.37.

9. A 30-year-old woman has had very itchy hands for 1 week. She has no previous history of skin disease. The rash is shown in Plate 7.38.

10. A 45-year-old man has had a painful rash on his right buttock only for 3 days. It is shown in Plate 7.39.

Causes of itchy painful rashes

For each patient with an itchy or painful rash, choose the *single* most likely diagnosis from the list of options below. Each option may be used once, more than once, or not at all. ★

A Bullous impetigo

B Bullous pemphigoid

C Dermatitis herpetiformis

D Lichen planus

E Pemphigus vulgaris

F Tinea capitis

G Tinea corporis

H Varicella zoster virus

11. A 28-year-old woman with hepatitis C has a very itchy rash over the volar aspect of her wrists, as shown in Plate 7.40. The rash also affects her ankles.

12. A 34-year-old man with coeliac disease has very itchy lesions over his buttocks, as shown in Plate 7.41. He has a similar rash over his elbows and knees.

13. A 75-year-old man has been itchy for 2 months. Over the past 2 weeks, he has developed lesions, as shown in Plate 7.42.

14. A 44-year-old man has painful blisters over his left arm, as shown in Plate 7.43. The remainder of his skin is unaffected.

15. A 67-year-old woman has eroded areas of skin on the trunk. Her mouth is very sore and has ulcers, as shown in Plate 7.44.

Causes of scaly rashes

For each patient, choose the *single* most likely diagnosis from the list of options below. Each option may be used once, more than once, or not at all. ★

A Atopic eczema

B Erythema multiforme

C Erythema nodosum

D Lichen planus

E Pityriasis rosea

F Pityriasis versicolor

G Psoriasis

H Tinea corporis

16. A 34-year-old man has a rash, as shown in Plate 7.45. He has had a similar rash for 20 years, but it has recently become much worse.

17. A 30-year-old woman has lesions over her trunk, palms, and soles, as shown in Plate 7.46. She had a cold sore on her lip the previous week.

18. A 12-year-old girl has non-itchy lesions on her arm, as shown in Plate 7.47. The rash started as a solitary lesion, but two more have since developed.

19. A 20-year-old woman has a scaly scalp, as shown in Plate 7.48. She also has scaly lesions over her elbows.

20. A 36-year-old woman has had an itchy rash for most of her life. It has been particularly severe over the past month. It is shown in Plate 7.49.

Drug treatments in skin disorders

For each patient with a rash, choose the *single* most appropriate treatment from the list of options below. Each option may be used once, more than once, or not at all. ★ ★

A Clobetasone butyrate

B Clobetasol propionate

C Ketoconazole shampoo

D Oral chlorphenamine

E Oral griseofulvin

F Oral non-steroidal anti-inflammatory drug

G Oral prednisolone

H Oral tetracycline

21. A 30-year-old woman has had a rash for 2 months. It is shown in Plate 7.50.

22. A 24-year-old woman is on the oral contraceptive pill, but no other medications. She has developed painful lumps on her shins, which are shown in Plate 7.51.

23. A 50-year-old man has had lesions on his face for 14 months, shown in Plate 7.52. He has tried potent topical corticosteroids, which helped initially, but then the spots became worse. The remainder of his skin is fine.

24. An 8-year-old girl has developed a boggy mass on her scalp, shown in Plate 7.53. For the past 3 months, she has had areas of hair loss that have been diagnosed as ringworm.

25. A 24-year-old man has tan-coloured patches on his trunk, which are shown in Plate 7.54. They appeared in the summer. They are not itchy.

Causes of hair and skin disorders

For each patient, choose the *single* most likely diagnosis from the list of options below. Each option may be used once, more than once, or not at all. ★ ★

A Acne keloidalis nuchae

B Alopecia areata

C Androgenetic alopecia

D Discoid lupus erythematosus

E Pityriasis alba

F Systemic lupus erythematosus

G Tinea capitis

H Vitiligo

26. A 38-year-old woman has noticed her hair thinning over the past year. Her thyroid function and ferritin levels are normal. Her scalp is shown in Plate 7.55.

27. A 33-year-old man has three discrete bald patches, one of which is shown in Plate 7.56. These have developed over the past 3 months. There has been no trauma to the scalp and he is otherwise well.

28. A 55-year-old woman has a patch of hair loss over the parietal region, shown in Plate 7.57. This has developed over the past 6 months. She also has atrophic erythematous plaques over her ears.

29. A 5-year-old boy has lost hair in patches over his scalp. This has progressed over the past 6 weeks and his scalp is shown in Plate 7.58.

30. A 25-year-old man has had a gradual loss of all of his hair. This started as two small bald patches, but has since spread to involve all of the hair on his head. He has also lost his eyebrows, eyelashes, and axillary hair. He is otherwise well and takes no medication. His scalp is shown in Plate 7.59.

ANSWERS

Single Best Answers

1. A ★   OHCS 8th edn → p589

This condition is more common in patients with type 2 diabetes. It causes velvety hyperpigmented plaques in the axillae, groin, and neck folds.

2. D ★   OHCS 8th edn → p596

This common dermatosis causes scaling and erythema in the nasolabial folds, eyebrows, and hairline. There may be associated fine scale on the scalp and within the ears.

3. D ★   OHCS 8th edn → p599

These are viral warts, caused by human papillomavirus

4. E ★   OHCS 8th edn → p584

5. B ★   OHCS 8th edn → p596

Atopic eczema is classically itchy. It typically affects flexural sites. It is common to get facial involvement, as seen here.

6. C ★   OHCS 8th edn → p599

This is eczema herpeticum (eczema infected with herpes simplex virus). Note the characteristic monomorphic vesicles. The history of the eczema getting worse despite antibiotics is a clue. This spreads very quickly and needs IV treatment.

7. D ★   OHCS 8th edn → p594

Note the symmetrical distribution of plaques with a silvery scale on the surface. The extensor aspects of the elbows are involved – a classical site for psoriasis.

8. B ★

This is neurofibromatosis type 1. It is an autosomal dominant condition. The multiple dome-shaped tumours are neurofibromas. There may also be café au lait macules and axillary freckling of the skin.
→ http://www.nfauk.org/ (The Neurofibromatosis Association)

9. C ★   OHCS 8th edn → p592

This is an acral subungual melanoma. Note the pigmentation of the skin around the nail (Hutchinson's sign). The nail has been distorted by the growth of the melanoma under the nail bed.

10. C ★   OHCS 8th edn → p594

The severe nail dystrophy, swollen distal interphalyngeal joints, and fine scaling over the fingertips are suggestive of psoriasis. Approximately 5% of patients with psoriasis develop arthropathy.

11. A ★

A patient with a hot red swollen leg may have cellulitis or a deep vein thrombosis. In this case, the raised temperature, the sharp demarcation of the erythema at the ankle, and the neutrophilia support the diagnosis of cellulitis.

12. D ★   OHCS 8th edn → p598

This is 'athlete's foot'. Note the macerated and scaled appearance of the skin in the web space.

13. A ★   OHCS 8th edn → p598

Impetigo can cause tense blisters, such as shown here. Note the yellow crusted patches, which are more typical of impetigo seen in children.

14. D ★   OHCS 8th edn → p584

The Köbner phenomenon describes skin lesions occurring in areas of trauma or surgery. It occurs with psoriasis (as seen here), warts, vitiligo, and lichen planus.

15. D ★   OHCS 8th edn → p592

Note the irregular colour and edge to this lesion. Remember the ABCDE for pigmented lesions:

Asymmetry
Border
Colour
Diameter >7mm
Evolution

16. A ★   OHCS 8th edn → p603

These are wheals. The history of them being present for less than 24h is typical. Acute urticaria can result from infection, drugs, or food allergy, but often no cause is found.

17. C ★   OHCS 8th edn → p588

The targetoid lesions are typical of erythema multiforme. This usually starts on the trunk and spreads acrally (to hands, feet, and head). Common causes are drugs and infection (typically herpes simplex virus or mycoplasma infection)

18. E ★   OHCS 8th edn → p602

Note the eroded areas from superficial blisters that have burst. This is typical of pemphigus vulgaris. The skin around the eroded areas is normal (unlike in bullous pemphigoid, when it is erythematous). The erosions on the lip further support the diagnosis of pemphigus vulgaris.

19. D ★   OHCS 8th edn → p588

This condition is more common in patients with inflammatory bowel disease. Note the ulcers with a purple–red border. The ulcers often appear undermined at the edge. Surgical intervention will make this condition worse and may lead to limb amputation – so don't cut these lesions out!

20. C ★   OHCS 8th edn → p590

This nodule is growing rapidly and has a symmetrical shape with a central plug of keratin. These lesions are usually excised in order to differentiate them from a squamous cell carcinoma.

21. E ★   OHCS 8th edn → p598

This is tinea corporis. It has been exacerbated by the topical steroid he has used. An oral antifungal is needed.

22. E ★   OHCS 8th edn → p590

This describes an exophytic tumour with a hyperkeratotic crust on a sun-exposed site. Squamous cell carcinoma is more common in organ-transplant recipients as a result of immunosuppressive medication, so must always be considered.

23. D ★   OHCS 8th edn → p600

For severe acne, isotretinoin for 16 weeks is the drug of choice. However, close supervision is required, as it has significant side effects.

24. E ★   OHCS 8th edn → p598

The satellite pustules visible are characteristic of candidiasis. The folds are involved (which makes an extrinsic dermatitis, such as irritant dermatitis, unlikely). This is treated with an antifungal cream such as nystatin.

25. B ★   OHCS 8th edn → p596

The distribution of this eruption gives the clue that this is allergic contact eczema – the eczema is limited to one body site. The face is a common site to be affected by allergic contact dermatitis (common allergens are make-up and hair dye).

26. D ★★   OHCS 8th edn → p600

This bulbous swelling of the nose has occurred as a result of long-standing rosacea. The tissues have been infiltrated by granulomatous inflammation.

27. D ★★

This is pompholyx hand eczema. It comprises very itchy vesicles and papules on the palms. Scabies is less likely here, because the papules come and go together with the rest of his eczema. This form of eczema requires treatment with a potent topical corticosteroid, such as betamethasone valerate.

28. B ★★   OHCS 8th edn → p586

The patches here have an indistinct border and are hypopigmented (not sharp-edged and depigmented, as would be seen in vitiligo). This is pityriasis alba, which occurs on faces of children with atopic eczema. It improves with emollients and mild topical corticosteroid creams.

29. A ★★   OHCS 8th edn → p602

Note the tense blisters on an erythematous, urticated base. Bullous pemphigoid does not usually affect the mucosal membranes.

30. D ★★   OHCS 8th edn → p588

This is a small-vessel vasculitis causing palpable purpura of the skin. This was caused by a hypersensitivity reaction to amoxicillin. Whenever purpura are seen, it is important to think of systemic sepsis; however, this man has too long a history and is well.

31. B ★★

This is melasma. The safest treatment is to advise the daily use of a sunblock. Sunshine makes this condition worse. Some women develop melasma while pregnant or when taking the oral contraceptive pill. Hydroquinone can be damaging to the skin, especially at high strength.

32. D ★★   OHCS 8th edn → p602

This is a benign vascular tumour that is more common in pregnancy. Lesions are often triggered by trauma.

33. D ★★

Note the tense blisters here. The surrounding skin is normal (which makes bullous pemphigoid, linear IgA disease, and allergic contact eczema unlikely). There is no evidence of impetigo here.

Extended Matching Questions

1. A ★

This glassy nodule has a rolled edge, typical of a basal cell carcinoma. The face is the commonest site to be affected by a basal cell carcinoma.

2. G ★

The warty surface of this plaque is typical of a seborrhoeic keratosis. Note the 'stuck-on' appearance.

3. D ★

This regular pink nodule has the characteristic 'button-hole' sign around the edge. Dermatofibromas commonly arise on the lower legs after an insect bite.

4. E ★

The history of this lesion increasing in size is a warning that this is a melanoma. The irregular, asymmetrical shape and edge with more than three different colours is highly suggestive of malignant melanoma.

5. B ★

This is a form of a birthmark that typically occurs at puberty. The shoulder is the characteristic site involved. A Becker's naevus often becomes more hairy with time.

General feedback on 1–5: OHCS 8th edn → pp590–592

6. G ★

This is cellulitis. It is caused by organisms that enter the body through a cut in the skin. It is important to take blood cultures and skin swabs. The other common organism that causes cellulitis is *Streptococcus*.

7. G ★

This is impetigo, which commonly starts around the nose and mouth, with a yellow crust on an erythematous base. It is most commonly caused by *Staphylococcus*. It is relatively common in children.

8. E ★

These are umbilicated papules in a cluster, typical of molluscum contagiosum virus infection. This is caused by a pox virus and is highly contagious.

9. F ★

This is scabies. The presence of itchy papules in the web spaces is characteristic of this condition. Burrows may also be seen.

10. H ★

This dermatomal collection of vesicles is characteristic of varicella-zoster virus infection (herpes zoster or shingles).

General feedback on 6–10: OHCS 8th edn → pp598–599

11. D ★

This is an inflammatory dermatosis that causes very itchy lichenoid papules (note the increased skin markings). Lichen planus is more common in patients infected with hepatitis C virus.

12. C ★

These extremely itchy vesiculopapular lesions affecting the extensor aspects are suggestive of dermatitis herpetiformis. This rash occurs in patients with gluten-sensitive enteropathy and the rash improves if a gluten-free diet is followed.

13. B ★

The tense dome-shaped blisters on an erythematous base are typical of bullous pemphigoid. This condition is more common in elderly patients. The itch often precedes the blisters.

14. H ★

The dermatomal distribution of the vesicles is the clue to this diagnosis.

15. E ★

Pemphigus vulgaris causes superficial blisters that burst easily, leaving erosions (compare with the deeper tense bullae in bullous pemphigoid). Pemphigus vulgaris commonly involves the mucosal membranes, including the mouth, causing erosions and ulcers.

General feedback on 11–15: OHCS 8th edn → pp588, 599, 602

16. G ★

Note the erythematous plaques with a silvery scale on the surface, affecting the extensor aspects of his body.

17. B ★

These are target lesions, seen in erythema multiforme. It is most commonly triggered by drugs or herpes simplex virus infection.

18. H ★

These are the characteristic annular scaly patches of ringworm (tinea corporis).

19. G ★

Psoriasis typically causes plaques over the extensor aspects of the body. It can also affect the scalp, nails, and joints.

20. A ★

Note the flexural distribution of scaly excoriated patches. This is severe eczema.

General feedback on 16–20: OHCS 8th edn →pp588, 594–597

21. H ★ ★

This is acne vulgaris. Note the multiple pustules. The most appropriate treatment is with a tetracycline drug.

22. F ★ ★

This is erythema nodosum. It was precipitated by the oral contraceptive pill. The appropriate treatment is rest and non-steroidal anti-inflammatory drugs (NSAIDs) and finding an alternative form of contraception.

23. H ★ ★

This is acne rosacea, made worse by topical corticosteroids. It is treated with oral tetracyclines for at least 4 months.

24. E ★ ★

This is a kerion, which occurs as part of the host's response to a fungal infection. It should be treated with an oral antifungal, such as griseofulvin or terbinafine, for at least 2 weeks. It should *not* be incised or drained.

25. C ★ ★

This is pityriasis versicolor, which is caused by a yeast infection on the skin surface. It is treated by using ketoconazole shampoo as a body wash for 1–2 weeks to stop scaliness. The pigmentation may take some time to recover. This condition often recurs.

26. C ★★

There is diffuse, non-scarring thinning of the hair. The scalp skin appears normal. This pattern of thinning over the vertex fits with the diagnosis of androgenetic alopecia in a female.

27. B ★★

There are focal patches of non-scarring alopecia. There are exclamation-mark hairs at the periphery (hairs that become narrower along the length of the strand closer to the base, producing a characteristic 'exclamation mark' appearance).

28. D ★★

This is a patch of scarring alopecia. Scarring alopecia can be caused by trauma, radiation, lichen planopilaris, and discoid lupus erythematosus. Atrophic plaques over the face or ears are characteristic of discoid lupus.

29. G ★★

This is the typical 'moth-eaten' appearance of tinea capitis. This would need treatment with a systemic antifungal agent, such as griseofulvin or terbinafine.

30. B ★★

This is alopecia areata universalis (loss of all body hair).

General feedback on 25–30: OHCS 8th edn →pp598, 602

Dermatology

CHAPTER 8

ANAESTHETICS AND CRITICAL CARE

Alex Bonner and James Dawson

Anaesthesia is a relatively young specialty when compared with its counterparts; William Morton gave the first anaesthetic in 1846 in Boston, Massachusetts. The Royal College of Anaesthetists was created from the Royal College of Surgeons in 1948, and anaesthetists now make up one of the largest groups of doctors by specialty.

Anaesthetists are highly trained physicians whose role is by no means limited to the operating theatre. Anaesthetists oversee the patient journey through the peri-operative period, which involves the pre-operative optimization of the sick patient, ensuring the safe induction, maintenance, and emergence from anaesthesia, and care of the patient in the early post-operative period. Anaesthetic skills are also requested in the Emergency Department with the critically ill and with the care of the parturient mother in providing analgesic, anaesthetic, and critical care services. Anaesthetists have an important role in the practice of Intensive Care, where complementary experience in medicine is useful. Other roles of the anaesthetist include provision of acute and chronic pain services, and subspecialty interests include regional, paediatric, cardiothoracic, and neuroanaesthesia.

Anaesthesia is a highly practical specialty, with a strong emphasis on the basic sciences underpinning its practice. Physiology and pharmacology exert their effects with immediacy, hence an affinity for these disciplines is desirable. Anaesthetists need to be able to assimilate knowledge of the basic sciences with skills in history and examination, in order to plan and respond to patient needs. In answering these questions, you will be asked to use similar skills. ∎

Alex Bonner

ANAESTHETICS AND CRITICAL CARE
SINGLE BEST ANSWERS

1. A 70-year-old man has had worsening shortness of breath for 2 days. He has a 50 pack year history of cigarette smoking, but otherwise has no previous medical history. He appears unwell, with a reduced level of consciousness and inadequate respiratory effort. The following arterial blood gas levels are obtained while breathing through a facemask with a reservoir bag, with an oxygen flow rate of 15L/min.

- pH 7.14
- pO_2 10.1kPa
- pCO_2 9.8kPa
- Bicarbonate 29.2mmol/L
- Base excess +9.4

Which is the single best description of the acid–base derangement? ★

A Metabolic acidosis with respiratory compensation

B Metabolic alkalosis with respiratory compensation

C Mixed respiratory and metabolic acidosis

D Respiratory acidosis with evidence of metabolic compensation

E Respiratory acidosis with no evidence of metabolic compensation

2. A 19-year-old man has fractured his right lower leg while playing football, about 30min ago. He was carried off the pitch on a stretcher. He is in discomfort and there is some blood staining on his sock. His right lower leg is immobilized in a box splint. He has an open fracture of his right distal tibia. There is no distal neurovascular deficit and he is haemodynamically stable; blood loss is estimated to be minimal. He has no other injuries and is fully alert. Which is the single most appropriate initial analgesia to give? ★

A IV morphine

B Oral codeine phosphate

C Oral gabapentin

D Oral paracetamol

E Rectal diclofenac

3. A 19-year-old woman is brought into the Emergency Department by paramedics. She was found unconscious in her bed by her parents, who also found empty packets of several prescription medications and a bottle of vodka. She does not open her eyes at all but withdraws to pain. She makes no verbal response. Which is her single Glasgow Coma Scale score? ★

A 3

B 6

C 9

D 12

E 15

4. A 56-year-old man has been thrombolysed for an anterior myocardial infarction 6h ago. His pain had eased but he suddenly has severe, central crushing chest pain radiating into his left arm. He becomes unconscious with no signs of life. The defibrillator is attached and the monitor shows the rhythm shown in Plate 8.1. Cardiopulomary resuscitation (CPR) with chest compressions and bag-valve-mask ventilation is started. He has IV access. Which is the single next most appropriate management? ★

A Continue CPR for 2min

B Defibrillation

C Endotracheal intubation

D IV atropine

E IV epinephrine (adrenaline)

5. A 24-year-old woman is having a procedure on her finger under ring block. Shortly after commencing, she feels light-headed and dizzy. She has ringing in her ears and tingling around the mouth. Which is the single most likely diagnosis? ★

A Acute labyrinthitis

B Anaphylaxis

C Failure of anaesthetic

D Local anaesthetic toxicity

E Vasovagal attack

6. A 34-year-old woman has been admitted to hospital with cellulitis of her forearm. She has just been given her second dose of IV penicillin. She now has chest tightness, difficulty in breathing, and feels dizzy. She has a diffuse urticarial rash all over her body and bilateral expiratory and inspiratory wheeze. Her pulse rate is 120bpm, her blood pressure is 80/40mmHg, and her oxygen saturation is 91% on room air. Which is the single most appropriate initial management? ★

A IM epinephrine (adrenaline) 0.5mg

B IV chlorphenamine 10mg

C IV epinephrine (adrenaline) 1mg

D IV hydrocortisone 100mg

E Take blood for serum mast cell tryptase

7. A 76-year-old woman had a left total knee replacement 4 days ago. She is normally fit and healthy. She has had an uncomplicated post-operative recovery, but the recent observations give her a Modified Early Warning Score of 6; it was 2 an hour ago. Her pulse rate is 120bpm, her blood pressure is 90/45mmHg, her oxygen saturation is 90% on room air, her respiratory rate is 30/min, and her temperature is 37.5°C. She is alert but has chest pain and shortness of breath. Which is the single most likely cause of her acute deterioration? ★

A Cardiac tamponade

B Myocardial infarction

C Pneumonia

D Pneumothorax

E Pulmonary embolism

8. A 24-year-old woman is 32 weeks pregnant with her first child. She has had pregnancy-induced hypertension. Her booking blood pressure was 125/76mmHg. She has come to the labour suite with a headache and she has some ankle oedema. Her blood pressure is now 145/92mmHg and urinalysis shows 3+ proteinuria. She suddenly loses consciousness and has a tonic–clonic seizure. She is put in the recovery position and given supplementary oxygen. She stops fitting and regains consciousness. Which is the single most appropriate next treatment? ★

A IV lorazepam

B IV magnesium sulphate

C IV phenytoin

D Oral methyldopa

E Sublingual nifedipine

9. A 19-year-old man has had a recurrent dislocation of his left shoulder. He has been given 20mg of IV midazolam and his shoulder is now reduced. He is now unconscious and has stopped breathing. Which is the single most appropriate immediate management? ★

A Connect ECG monitoring

B Give IV flumazenil

C Give IV naloxone

D Intubate the patient

E Open the airway with a jaw thrust

10. A 63-year-old woman had a redo total hip replacement under general anaesthetic 3 days ago. She has chest pain, which developed suddenly and is worse on inspiration. Her pulse rate is 110bpm, her oxygen saturation is 90% on 5L of oxygen by mask, and her temperature is 37.4°C. Which single investigation is likely to confirm the diagnosis? ★

A Chest X-ray

B CT pulmonary angiogram

C ECG

D Echocardiography

E Cardiac enzymes

11. A 64-year-old woman had an inferior myocardial infarction (MI) 12h ago. She has been successfully thrombolysed. She suddenly develops a profound narrow complex bradycardia with a rate of 30bpm. Her blood pressure is 75/39mmHg and she feels dizzy and sick. Which is the single most appropriate immediate management? ★

A IV amiodarone

B IV atropine

C IV isoprenaline

D Transcutaneous (external) cardiac pacing

E Transvenous cardiac pacing

12. A 6-week-old boy, who was born prematurely, has had vomiting and lethargy for 5 days. He has sunken eyes and reduced skin turgor. His capillary refill time is 4s. The following arterial blood gas sample is obtained.

- pH 7.52
- P_aCO_2 5.0kPa.
- P_aO_2 11.0kPa.
- HCO_3 34.2mmol/L
- Base excess +9.1

Which is the single best description of his metabolic status? ★

A Metabolic acidosis without respiratory compensation

B Metabolic alkalosis with respiratory compensation

C Metabolic alkalosis without respiratory compensation

D Respiratory alkalosis with metabolic compensation

E Respiratory alkalosis without metabolic compensation

13. A 68-year-old man has chronic obstructive pulmonary disease (COPD). He has been involved in a motor vehicle collision. He has a fractured femur and signs of a tension pneumothorax. His oxygen saturation is 76% on room air and his arterial blood gas shows:

- pH 7.5
- pO_2 4.5 kPa
- pCO_2 3.5 kPa
- Bicarbonate 32mmol/L

He is being prepared for a needle thoracocentesis. Which is the single most appropriate means of oxygen delivery to use? ★

A Face-mask continuous positive airway pressure (CPAP)

B Immediate intubation and ventilation

C Nasal cannulae

D Non-rebreathe mask with reservoir bag

E Venturi mask with 35% oxygen delivery

14. A 20-year-old man is undergoing his first ever general anaesthetic for an elective tonsillectomy. Shortly after administration of the induction agents, he becomes unwell. Which is the single most likely first sign indicating that he may be having an anaphylactic reaction?★

A Angio-oedema

B Cough

C Desaturation

D Hypotension

E Rash

15. A 35-year-old man is seen on the day-case unit prior to an arthroscopy for knee pain. He describes himself as 'fit and well' and does not smoke. He takes inhalers for asthma, which is well controlled, and has no other medical problems. Which single ASA (American Society of Anesthesiologists) grade best describe his physical status?★ ★

A I

B II

C III

D IV

E V

16. A 31-year-old woman is scheduled for an elective laparoscopic cholecystectomy. After intubation, the CO_2 (capnography) trace diminishes, she begins to desaturate, and the anaesthetist is unable to hear air entry when auscultating over the chest, despite being able to hand ventilate her easily. Which is the single most likely cause for this? ★ ★

A Anaphylaxis

B Cardiac arrest

C Monitoring failure

D Oesophageal intubation

E Bilateral pneumothoraces

17. Urgent help is required in the anaesthetic room. A patient has become rapidly unwell at induction of anaesthesia. He has generalized muscle rigidity and tachycardia, and appears sweaty. His blood pressure is normal. Which is the single most likely diagnosis? ★ ★

A Acute dystonia

B Anaphylaxis

C Epileptic seizure

D Malignant hyperthermia

E Suxamethonium apnoea

18. A 49-year-old woman has presumed sepsis arising from her biliary tract. She is known to have hypertension and gall stones. The admitting team have obtained IV access and taken blood. She has also received a dose of broad-spectrum antibiotics. Her blood pressure is 91/40mmHg and her serum lactate is 3.6mmol/L. Which is the single most important next management step, according to the Surviving Sepsis Campaign (2008)? ★ ★

A Commence a vasopressor infusion

B Give a minimum 20ml/kg fluid bolus

C Insert a peripheral arterial line

D Insert a central venous catheter

E Re-check serum lactate

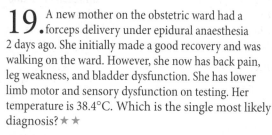

19. A new mother on the obstetric ward had a forceps delivery under epidural anaesthesia 2 days ago. She initially made a good recovery and was walking on the ward. However, she now has back pain, leg weakness, and bladder dysfunction. She has lower limb motor and sensory dysfunction on testing. Her temperature is 38.4°C. Which is the single most likely diagnosis? ★ ★

A Bacterial meningitis

B Brown-Séquard syndrome

C Peroneal nerve palsy

D Prolapsed intervertebral disc

E Spinal abscess

20. A previously fit and well 34-year-old man is undergoing surgery for a fractured right femur. He is under a general anaesthetic and the orthopaedic surgeons have just inserted the femoral nail. Intra-operative blood loss is estimated to be about 2000mL. He has been given 3000mL of IV fluid throughout the operation. A bedside haemoglobin test gives a haemoglobin level of 6.9g/dL. His pulse rate is 90bpm and his blood pressure is 125/75mmHg. No further blood loss is anticipated. Which is the single most appropriate next step in management? ★ ★

A Administration of recombinant activated factor VIIa

B Prescribe post-operative iron tablets

C Transfusion of fully cross-matched blood

D Transfusion of group O rhesus-negative blood

E Transfusion of group-specific blood

21. A 53-year-old woman returns to recovery after a laparoscopic cholecystectomy. The procedure was technically difficult and lasted longer than anticipated. Her temperature in recovery is 32.9°C. Which single physical process accounts for the greatest heat loss intra-operatively? ★ ★

A Conduction

B Convection

C Humidification

D Radiation

E Respiration

22. A 31-year-old man has sustained a cut to his right (dominant) hand while at work. The cut is on the palm of the hand on the radial aspect. A median nerve block at the wrist is planned to provide sufficient anaesthesia for the wound to be explored and sutured. Which single option describes where the median nerve lies at the wrist? ★ ★

A Between the tendons of the palmaris longus and the flexor pollicis longus

B Lateral to the radial artery

C Medial to the ulnar artery

D Medial to the ulnar nerve

E Superficial to the flexor retinaculum

23. A 17-year-old man has HbAS (sickle cell trait). He is having repair of a fractured radius under general anaesthetic. During the procedure, the surgeon uses a tourniquet to create a bloodless field, and K-wires the fracture. The patient receives IV fluids, analgesia, and post-operatively is given oxygen. Which single factor is associated with an increased risk of sickle cell crisis? ★ ★

A IV fluid therapy

B Opioid analgesia

C Oxygen therapy

D Prophylactic antibiotics

E Tourniquet use

24. An 82-year-old man undergoes a transurethral resection of the prostate (TURP) procedure under spinal anaesthetic. The procedure was long and the surgeon required large volumes of irrigating fluid. In recovery, he becomes increasingly agitated and confused, his Glasgow Coma Scale score falls, and he needs intubation. Which is the single most likely metabolic abnormality to account for this? ★ ★

A Hyperglycaemia

B Hypernatraemia

C Hypoglycaemia

D Hypokalaemia

E Hyponatraemia

25. A 42-year-old woman had a partial thyroidectomy 24h ago. Her pre-operative haemoglobin level was 11.4g/dL. Today's result is 3.8g/dL. She is pain free, her pulse rate is 85bpm, and her blood pressure is 118/76mmHg. Blood loss was estimated to be about 300mL and there is minimal fluid in the surgical drain. Her neck is not distended and the wound site is clean and dry. Which is the single most likely cause of the anaemia? ★ ★ ★

A Bone marrow failure

B Iron deficiency

C Major intra-operative haemorrhage

D Ongoing post-operative haemorrhage

E Spurious result

26. A 29-year-old man has been on the Intensive Therapy Unit for 2 days following a serious motor vehicle collision. He is making no respiratory effort and tests show that he has brainstem death. The medical team is planning to talk to the relatives about the possibility of organ donation. Which single advice is correct in relation to organ donation? ★ ★ ★ ★

A Organs can only be harvested once the donor's heart has stopped beating

B Organ donation can only take place if the donor is on the organ donor register or carried an organ donation card

C Organs of patients who are human immunodeficiency virus (HIV) positive are usually taken

D Organs will usually be harvested if the donor is on the organ donation register, even if the next of kin do not wish for organ donation

E The next of kin can specify if they do not want particular organs to be donated

27. A 35-year-old woman is undergoing a diagnostic laparoscopy for pelvic pain. She is deemed to be at high risk for post-operative nausea and vomiting. Which single class of drugs can be used in the prophylaxis of post-operative nausea and vomiting? ★ ★ ★ ★

A Anticonvulsants

B Benzodiazepines

C Corticosteroids

D Opioids

E Smooth muscle relaxants

28. An 80-year-old woman is undergoing palliative care for inoperable cancer. She has copious secretions in the upper airway that are troublesome and is requesting something to help. Which single group of drugs is the most appropriate to prescribe? ★ ★ ★ ★

A Acetylcholinesterase inhibitors

B Anticholinergics

C Antihistamines

D Dopamine antagonists

E Sympathomimetics

EXTENDED MATCHING QUESTIONS

Causes of poisoning

For each patient, choose the *single* most likely diagnosis from the list of options below. Each option may be used once, more than once, or not at all. ★

A Alcohol poisoning

B Amitriptyline overdose

C Benzodiazepine overdose

D Beta-blocker overdose

E Carbamazepine overdose

F Carbon monoxide poisoning

G Digoxin toxicity

H Lithium overdose

I Opioid overdose

J Oxygen toxicity

K Paracetamol overdose

L Paraquat poisoning

1. A young man has been found unresponsive on a street corner. His airway is being maintained with an oropharyngeal airway device and a jaw thrust, and he is making infrequent and shallow breaths. He has pin-point pupils. His pulse rate is 70bpm, his blood pressure is 90/50mmHg, and his Glasgow Coma Scale score is 3/15.

2. A 19-year-old woman has abdominal pain and vomiting. She took an overdose of tablets two nights ago while drunk, but is not sure what the tablets were. She has right upper-quadrant tenderness. Her pulse rate is 100bpm, her blood pressure is 102/59mmHg, and her Glasgow Coma Scale score is 15/15. Blood tests show:
- Bilirubin 100 µmol/L
- Alanine aminotransferase 780IU/L
- International normalized ratio (INR) 5.0

3. A 21-year-old woman has taken an overdose of her mother's prescription tablets. She is pale and clammy. Her pulse rate is 30bpm and her blood pressure is 75/33mmHg. An ECG shows a profound sinus bradycardia.

4. A 59-year-old man has been found in his car in a remote location, by the police. He was initially unresponsive. In the Emergency Department, he is drowsy and confused. He is very pink in colour. His pulse rate is 90bpm, his blood pressure 110/50mmHg, and his oxygen saturation on finger probe is 100% on high-flow oxygen.

5. A 78-year-old man has mistakenly taken too many of his regular tablets. He is vomiting and mildly confused. He says everything looks yellow. His pulse rate is 40bpm and his blood pressure is 90/43mmHg. An ECG shows very slow atrial fibrillation.

Drugs used in emergencies

For each patient, choose the *single* most appropriate initial management from the list of options below. Each option may be used once, more than once, or not at all. ★ ★ ★

A Adenosine 3mg IV

B Amiodarone 300mg IV

C Atropine 2–3mg IV

D Calcium gluconate 10% 10mL IV

E Calcium resonium 30g per rectum

F Chlorpheniramine 10mg IV

G Diazepam 30mg per rectum

H Epinephrine (adrenaline) 0.5mg IV

I Epinephrine 0.5mg IM

J Epinephrine 1mg IV

K Epinephrine 1mg IM

L Glucagon 1mg IV

M Hydrocortisone 200mg IV

N Lorazepam 4mg IV

O Magnesium sulphate 1.2–2g IV

P Potassium chloride 20 mmol

Q Prednisolone 30mg oral

R Salbutamol 3–20 mg/min IV infusion

S Salbutamol 5mg nebulized

T Sodium bicarbonate 8.4% 50mL IV

6. A 21-year-old man is brought into the resuscitation room following a motor vehicle collision. During the primary survey, his central pulse is lost and cardiopulmonary resuscitation is commenced. The pads are attached and the monitor shows pulseless electrical activity at a rate of 80bpm.

7. A 24-year-old man has had a severe reaction to peanuts. He is cyanotic, wheezy, and covered in an urticarial rash. His blood pressure is 85/60 mmHg.

8. A 30-year-old man with asthma has a peak expiratory flow rate of <33% of predicted. His respiratory rate is 26/min and his pulse rate is 115bpm. Oxygen is given at 15 L/min via a facemask with reservoir bag.

9. A 45-year-old man has had profuse watery diarrhoea and vomiting for 5 days. He has not been able to tolerate oral fluids and is profoundly dehydrated. While the results of his blood tests are awaited, an ECG is performed, which shows tall tented T waves, flattening of P waves, and widening of the QRS complexes.

10. A 61-year-old man with a history of depression and self-harm is brought into the Emergency Department. He has ingested a large volume of commercial pesticide. He is wheezy and has excessive salivation and lacrimation. He has diarrhoea and his pupils are meiotic. His heart rate is 60bpm.

Single Best Answers

1. D ★

The blood gas shows a marked respiratory acidosis. As is common in patients with smoking-related lung disease, a degree of metabolic compensation for a chronically elevated pCO_2 occurs, shown by the raised bicarbonate level. However, this man is unwell with a grossly elevated pCO_2, exceeding the buffering capacity of the blood. He has a reduced level of consciousness from CO_2 narcosis.

The flow chart below sets out a step-by-step guide on how to approach blood gases:

ACIDOSIS: pH <7.35	ALKALOSIS: pH >7.45
Look at the base excess first:	Look at the base excess first.
Normal (−3 to +3) = **respiratory acidosis** and pCO_2 will be raised (>6kPa)	Normal (−3 to +3) = **respiratory alkalosis** and pCO_2 will be low (<4.5kPa)
High negative (>−4) = **metabolic acidosis**. If pCO_2 is normal (4.5–6kPa), it is just a metabolic acidosis. If pCO_2 is low (<4.5kPa), there is **respiratory compensation**. If the pCO_2 is also high, it is a **mixed acidosis**.	High positive (>+4) = **metabolic alkalosis**. If pCO_2 is normal (4.5–6kPa) it is just a metabolic alkalosis, if pCO_2 is high (>6kPa) there is **respiratory compensation**, if pCO_2 is low then it is a **mixed alkalosis**.
High positive (>+4) = **respiratory acidosis with renal compensation**. The pCO_2 will be high (>6kPa).	High negative (>−4) = **respiratory alkalosis with renal compensation**. The pCO_2 will be low (<4.5kPa).

2. A ★   OHCS 8th edn → p636

Acute severe pain is best managed with strong opioids, such as morphine and diamorphine. Common routes of administration of the strong opioids in acute pain include IV, oral, intra-nasal, and subcutaneous. IV administration will provide the most rapid pain relief and avoid first-pass metabolism by the liver; first-pass metabolism mostly affects orally administered drugs. The strong opioids should be titrated to effect.

The World Health Organization (WHO) analgesic ladder offers a step-wise approach to pain management, although the severity of acute pain needs to be assessed to ensure that treatment begins on the appropriate 'rung' of the ladder.

Treating this patient with oral paracetamol or a weak opioid alone would be insufficient for his acute pain. Combining a strong opioid with paracetamol and a non-steroidal anti-inflammatory drug (such as diclofenac or ibuprofen) will reduce the overall amount of opioid needed to control his pain. This is beneficial, as it will minimize the risk of opioid side effects (sedation, nausea and vomiting, constipation, etc).

→ http://www.ganfyd.org/images/thumb/7/77/WHO_Analgesic_Ladder.png/550px-WHO_Analgesic_Ladder.png

3. B ★   OHCS 8th edn → p720

The Glasgow Coma Scale (GCS) is used to assess and record the level of consciousness of a patient. Although developed for use on the traumatized patient, GCS assessment is used on virtually all patients who present with a depressed level of consciousness, irrespective of the cause.

Best eye response	Score
No eye opening	1
Eyes open to pain	2
Eyes open to command	3
Eyes open spontaneously	4
Best motor response	
No motor response	1
Extensor posturing to pain	2
Abnormal flexor posturing to pain	3
Withdraws to pain (normal flexion)	4
Localizing response to pain	5
Obeys command	6

Best verbal response	
No sounds	1
Incomprehensible sound	2
Inappropriate speech	3
Confused conversation	4
Normal	5

4. B ★

This man is in ventricular fibrillation (VF) and requires immediate electrical defibrillation. The fibrillating heart has electrical activity but this is unco-ordinated and the heart cannot function as a pump. Passing electricity through the heart (defibrillation) causes transient cessation of all endogenous electrical activity. Once this happens, the intrinsic pacemakers should take over and result again in co-ordinated contractions of the atria and ventricles.

Chest compressions alone are very unlikely to cardiovert VF into a perfusing rhythm, and if a defibrillator is immediately available, a defibrillating shock should be given as soon as VF is identified. Once VF is identified, the initial shock takes precedence over airway, breathing, and the administration of any drugs.

The step-wise management of VF and pulseless ventricular tachycardia (VT) are the same and are outlined in the Adult Advanced Life Support Algorithm.
→ http://www.resus.org.uk/pages/als.pdf

5. D ★   OHCS 8th edn → p632

Whenever local anaesthetic is used, the possibility of toxicity should be considered. Even with relatively small doses, inadvertent rapid intravascular injection of anaesthetic can result in toxicity. The first symptoms of local anaesthetic toxicity are due to central nervous system (CNS) stimulation (tinnitus, circumoral paraesthesia, light-headedness, and dizziness), followed by CNS depression leading to cardiovascular system depression. If a patient complains of symptoms suggestive of toxicity, the operator should immediately stop injecting anaesthetic.

6. A ★

This patient is having an anaphylactic reaction, probably secondary to antibiotics. The priorities in management should follow the Airway, Breathing, Circulation approach – see the Adult Advanced Life Support algorithm.

If anaphylaxis is suspected, the precipitant should be stopped (e.g. stop antibiotic infusion) and the patient given IM epinephrine 0.5mg (0.5mL of 1:1000 epinephrine). It is unlikely that IM epinephrine will cause an adverse event if it later transpires that the patient was not having an anaphylactic reaction. If in doubt, give the IM epinephrine.

Chlorphenamine, hydrocortisone, and taking blood for mast cell tryptase are all indicated in cases of anaphylaxis, but epinephrine takes priority.
→ http://www.resus.org.uk/pages/anaalgo.pdf

7. E ★

This woman has had lower-limb surgery and is likely to have been fairly immobile for the last 4 days. She is at high risk of a deep vein thrombosis and subsequent pulmonary embolism. This is the most likely pathology.

Beck's triad (muffled heart sounds, raised jugular venous pressure, and hypotension) would make cardiac tamponade more likely, but this is not pathognomonic. Equally, there is no history of ischaemic heart disease, and an acute myocardial infarction is unlikely to give rise to desaturation unless there was gross heart failure. Pneumonia is relatively common in the post-operative population, but usually has a more gradual onset of cough, pyrexia, anorexia, and lethargy. Pneumothoraces can be rapid in onset, but again there is no reason here to suggest that she is at risk from this (such as pre-existing lung disease, positive pressure ventilation, central lines, etc).

The Modified Early Warning Score is an objective way of monitoring patients for deterioration:

Total score	Action
2	Repeat observations in 30min
3	Inform junior doctor
>4	Request junior doctor immediately

The Modified Early Warning Score (MEWS) is calculated as follows:

	3	2	1	0	1	2	3
Respiratory rate (breaths/min)		<9		9–14	15–20	21–29	>30
Heart rate (bpm)		<40	41–50	51–100	101–110	111–129	>130
Systolic BP (mmHg)	<70	71–80	81–100	101–199		>200	
Temperature (°C)		<35		35–38.4		>38.5	
AVPU				<u>A</u>lert	Reacts to <u>V</u>oice	Reacts to <u>P</u>ain	<u>U</u>nresponsive

→ http://www.gp-training.net/protocol/cardiovascular/dvt.htm
→ http://qjmed.oxfordjournals.org/cgi/content/full/94/10/521

8. B ★

This patient initially had pre-eclampsia. Pre-eclampsia is diagnosed after 20 weeks' gestation when there is hypertension (systolic blood pressure (BP) >140mmHg and/or diastolic BP >90mmHg) or a rise in systolic BP of >30mmHg or a rise in diastolic BP of >15mmHg compared with the booking BP, and greater than 300mg/dL per 24h of protein in the urine. Eclampsia is when a patient with pre-eclampsia has a seizure.

The Magpie Trial (*Lancet* 360:1331, 2002) demonstrated that patients with pre-eclampsia were less likely to go on to eclampsia if they were given IV magnesium. This and other work has also formed the basis on which the first-line treatment for eclampsia is IV magnesium.
→ http://emedicine.medscape.com/article/261435-overview

9. E ★

This patient has respiratory depression secondary to benzodiazepine excess. The immediate approach to any critically ill patient begins with airway assessment and treatment of any problems with it. This must take place before moving on to breathing and then on to circulation; this is outlined in the Adult Advanced Life Support algorithm. If the patient's airway in not patent or safe after a jaw thrust and use of airway adjuncts (e.g. Guedel airway), then they will need intubation. Applying ECG leads is part of the assessment of the circulation.

Naloxone is the reversal agent used in opioid overdose. Flumazenil is the reversal agent in benzodiazepine overdose, but again airway takes precedence over flumazenil in this case.
→ http://www.resus.org.uk/pages/als.pdf

10. B ★

This history points towards the diagnosis of pulmonary embolism in the post-operative period. Pelvic and orthopaedic surgery are risk factors for pulmonary embolism. Whilst chest X-ray and ECG may point towards pulmonary embolism, CT pulmonary angiography is the investigation of choice in most hospitals to confirm the diagnosis.

11. B ★

This patient has a bradycardia, which is probably secondary to her inferior MI and which is causing cardiovascular compromise (hypotension). In accordance with the Adult Bradycardia Algorithm, she has adverse signs of her bradycardia and the first-line treatment should be with IV atropine (an anticholinergic). Should the bradycardia persist, then IV isoprenaline (a β-adrenoceptor agonist), transcutaneous (external), and transvenous cardiac pacing may all be utilized.

Amiodarone is used to treat tachyarrhythmias and often results in bradycardia.
→ http://www.resus.org.uk/pages/bradalgo.pdf

12. C ★ OHCS 8th edn → p172

A child with pyloric stenosis classically presents with a metabolic alkalosis due to loss of acid from the upper gastrointestinal tract. A flow chart giving a step-by-step guide on how to approach blood gases in given in the answer to question 1.

13. D ★

This man's tension pneumothorax is life-threatening. He also needs a high concentration of oxygen delivered to his functioning lung as he is grossly hypoxaemic. The concern is that a patient with COPD potentially has a 'hypoxic drive' and that giving oxygen will cause the patient to hypoventilate, retain CO_2, and become drowsy. This is not a concern in this life-threatening emergency setting; the patient is likely to die of hypoxaemia or circulatory collapse secondary to the tension pneumothorax first, unless treated. The O_2 concentration can be reduced once the patient is more stable.

A face mask with a non-rebreathe valve and reservoir bag will deliver about 80% O_2 when the O_2 is turned on to 15L/min. Nasal cannulae will deliver about 28% and the Venturi system will deliver 35%, both of which are insufficient in this setting. Face-mask CPAP is likely to expand this pneumothorax further, as would intubation and ventilation — a chest drain must be sited before commencing either of these in this situation.

14. D ★   OHCS 8th edn → p237

→ http://www.aagbi.org/publications/guidelines/docs/anaphylaxis03.pdf

15. B ★★   OHCS 8th edn → p615

Class II refers to a patient with a mild systemic disease. The ASA grading of patient status was introduced in the 1960s. Although simple, it has been shown to correlate with the risks associated with anaesthesia and surgery, and therefore forms part of the pre-operative assessment of all patients undergoing general anaesthesia.

ASA grade	Description	Mortality rate (%)
I	Normally healthy individual	0.1
II	Patient with mild systemic disease	0.2
III	Patient with severe systemic disease that is not incapacitating	1.8
IV	Patient with incapacitating systemic disease that is a constant threat to life	7.8
V	Moribund patient who is not expected to survive 24h with or without an operation	9.4

The mortality rates quoted are an average for both elective and emergency surgery. The suffix E is added to denote an emergency operation.

16. D ★★   OHCS 8th edition → p627

Anaphylaxis usually presents with a combination of bronchospasm, rash, tachycardia, and hypotension; as the patient is easy to hand ventilate, this is unlikely as bronchospastic lungs require high airway pressures.

Cardiac arrest would cause an absent pulse oximetry trace, and breath sounds would still be audible while she is being hand ventilated.

A failure of monitoring equipment is unlikely to give this picture, as both the capnography and the pulse oximetry modules would have to be faulty at the same time and she may well become cyanotic.

Bilateral pneumothoraces would be very unlucky, but could give rise to this situation. Probability dictates that this is very unlikely.

Oesophageal intubation is the most likely cause here, and could be confirmed by auscultating over the stomach and hearing borborygmi when hand ventilating the patient. Its management involves removal of the misplaced tube, re-oxygenating the patient with mask ventilation, and then intubating the trachea.

17. D ★ ★ OHCS 8th edn → p628

Malignant hyperthermia is an inherited disorder of calcium metabolism affecting skeletal muscle. It is most often triggered by suxamethonium or the volatile anaesthetic agents. Its presentation varies from individual to individual, but should be considered where there is unexplained tachycardia, especially in the presence of tachypnoea, muscle rigidity, or an increase in end-tidal pCO_2. Malignant hyperthermia requires urgent management, which includes removal of the trigger agent, cooling, and treatment with dantrolene. Without treatment, mortality is approximately 75%; with treatment, mortality is significantly lowered.

None of the other diagnoses classically present as described. Acute dystonia is often triggered by neuroleptic agents, and typically presents in the first few days of new treatment. It is very rarely associated with anaesthesia. Suxamethonium apnoea is an inherited deficiency in plasma cholinesterase, resulting is delayed metabolism of suxamethonium and therefore prolongation of neuromuscular blockade.

18. B ★ ★

Vasoactive mediators from the infective agent and from damaged endothelium are causing widespread vasodilatation, hypotension, and a resultant tachycardia. The goals in managing septic shock are firstly to ensure adequate filling (pre-load), as measured by the central venous pressure (CVP). Once the patient is adequately filled, if hypotension and shock persist, a vasopressor should then be commenced, such as noradrenaline (norepinephrine; acting predominantly upon α_1-adrenoceptors).

A central line will allow the CVP to be measured, but more important than the specific value recorded is the trend in pressure in response to fluid boluses; if the CVP continues to rise, this usually suggests that more fluid is needed, whereas a plateau in the CVP suggests adequate filling has been achieved. A central line will also allow some drugs to be administered that are otherwise irritant to smaller peripheral veins.

An arterial line will be useful in the High-Dependency Unit/Intensive Therapy Unit setting but is not a priority in the first instance. Similarly, re-checking the serum lactate is unlikely to be of use within the first 6h.
→ http://www.survivingsepsis.org/6hr_bundles

19. E ★★

The history points to a rare but documented complication of spinal and epidural anaesthesia. The examination findings, supported by the presence of fever, point towards this diagnosis.

20. C ★★

Losing more than 20% of the circulating volume is regarded as a significant blood loss and in most circumstances this needs to be replaced with a blood transfusion. Circulating volume is approximately 70mL/kg, so around 4900mL in a 70kg man. As this patient is haemodynamically stable, there is no urgency for this, so there is time to obtain fully cross-matched blood, which usually takes about 45min to become available; this blood will be thoroughly matched for his blood group (A, B, AB, or O), rhesus D status (negative or positive) and for rarer antibodies/antigens. Type-specific blood takes about 20min to be available and is matched only for blood group and rhesus D status, but not for the rarer antibodies/antigens. Group O rhesus-negative blood, the universal donor, should be available immediately in most clinical areas, but carries the risk of the patient raising antibodies to the rarer antigens, which can cause problems with future blood transfusions. The decision about which blood to request depends upon the clinical urgency.

The link below is to the National Blood Service website and shows the current stocks of blood.
→ http://www.blood.co.uk/StockGraph/stocklevelstandard.aspx

21. D ★★   OHCS 8th edn → p628

Radiation accounts for approximately 40% of the heat lost from the body. Convection (30%), respiration (including humidification) (20%), and conduction (10%) are all important and their relative contributions vary depending on the environment. Space blankets are designed to reduce heat loss from radiation.

22. A ★ ★   OHCS 8th edn → p761

The median nerve lies between the two prominent tendons at the wrist (palmaris longus and flexor pollicis longus) and is deep to the flexor retinaculum within the carpal tunnel. Swelling within the carpal tunnel gives rise to 'carpal tunnel syndrome' caused by compression upon the median nerve.

The ulna bone, ulnar nerve, and ulnar artery are medial to the median nerve, and the radial artery lies lateral to it.

23. E ★ ★

Use of a tourniquet is associated with precipitation of sickle cell crisis. All of the other options are associated with minimizing the risk of a crisis and should form part of the peri-operative care where appropriate.

24. E ★ ★

TURP syndrome is a complication of TURP and is caused by the combination of fluid overload and hyponatraemia. It can be complicated by hyperglycinaemia (not hyperglycaemia) as a result of the glycine irrigation fluid that is used by the surgeons. Hence, the mental state of patients should be regularly assessed peri-operatively, and any sign of confusion should be a cause for concern. Long procedures are a risk factor for TURP syndrome. Management consists of slow correction of the underlying metabolic disturbance.

25. E ★ ★ ★

There is no suggestion that there was significant intra-operative or post-operative bleeding so major blood loss is unlikely. Iron-deficiency anaemia is a chronic pathology and would take longer than 24h to develop. Bone marrow failure can result in anaemia, but is relatively rare and usually causes a pancytopenia, so it would be important to check the platelet and white cell counts too. Most importantly, this patient has no features of profound anaemia such as circulatory collapse (shock).

The most likely cause is a spurious result from either an error when taking the blood sample (such as taking it from the drip arm and causing dilution) or from a laboratory error (much less likely). As there are no features of circulatory compromise, a new sample should be taken and analysed.

→ http://www.surgical-tutor.org.uk/default-home.htm?core/preop1/anaemia.htm~right

26. E ★ ★ ★ ★   OHCS 8th edn → p777

The majority of organ donations in the UK occur from heart-beating donors. The use of non-heart-beating donors is increasing in the UK, but this is still relatively uncommon. A patient does not have to be registered on the organ donor register to donate organs, but if they expressed that they would not want to donate organs during life, then this decision is usually honoured. If a patient had expressed that they wanted to donate their organs but their living next of kin was against organ donation, then it is unlikely that organs would be taken, as this would go against the relatives' wishes.

→ https://www.uktransplant.org.uk

27. C ★ ★ ★ ★

Dexamethasone, a corticosteroid, 4–8mg IV, is commonly used as an anti-emetic. It is usually given intraoperatively, as is associated with unpleasant side effects when given to the awake patient.

28. B ★ ★ ★ ★

Anticholinergics, e.g. hyoscine, are routinely used for their antisialogogue effect, particularly in the palliative care setting. Acetylcholine is the neurotransmitter at muscarinic receptors of the parasympathetic nervous system, responsible for control of secretions. Hence, anticholinergic drugs will block this pathway.

Extended Matching Questions

1. I ★

The combination of pin-point pupils and shallow and sighing infrequent respiration should alert you to opioid overdose.

2. D ★

Beta-blockers inhibit epinephrine (adrenaline)-mediated sympathetic effects on the heart and blood vessels and cause severe bradycardia and hypotension in overdose.

3. K ★

This is the most common overdose seen acutely. Delayed presentation can cause potentially fatal liver damage, and the risk is worsened by concurrent alcohol consumption. Paracetamol hepatotoxicity is the commonest cause of acute liver failure in the UK.

4. F ★

Carbon monoxide (CO) toxicity can easily be missed as patients appear pink and have oxygen saturations of 100% peripherally, due to the presence of carboxyhaemoglobin. CO has a significant affinity for haemoglobin and also affects the release of oxygen to the tissues. With a suspicious history, such as this, carboxyhaemoglobin levels must be measured.

5. G ★

Digoxin has a low therapeutic index and toxicity is common, especially in the elderly. Yellow vision (xanthopsia) is characteristic, along with nausea, anorexia, and confusion. Various ECG changes can occur.

6. J ★★★

→ http://www.resus.org.uk/pages/als.pdf

7. I ★★★

→ http://www.resus.org.uk/pages/reaction.pdf#search="anaphylaxis"

8. S ★★★

9. D ★★★

The ECG signs indicate hyperkalaemia. The priority is to give a cardioprotective agent, calcium gluconate.

10. C ★★★

This is the presentation of organophosphate poisoning, which classically presents with signs of a cholinergic syndrome, and is treated with atropine and pralidoxime.

CHAPTER 9
TRAUMA AND ORTHOPAEDICS

Nev Davies

O ver the years, trauma and orthopaedics has evolved into a vast specialty that is ever growing, with new technology, techniques, and implants. Computer-assisted surgery and minimally invasive approaches are current hot topics that are pushing the boundaries of delivering the best possible care for patients.

This specialty touches people of all ages from all walks of life. The practicality and logic in decision-making and management appeals to today's modern 'orthopods'.

Trauma is a team specialty, and orthopaedic surgeons play an essential role in the initial and definitive management of patients with musculoskeletal injuries, saving life and saving limb.

Paediatric orthopaedics is a highly specialized area. However, as a doctor in any setting, it is invaluable to have an understanding of the presentation of common children's orthopaedic conditions, such as developmental dysplasia of the hip and septic arthritis, which, if unrecognized, can have serious consequences for the rest of the child's life.

Arthroplasty has been one of the true successes of the 21st century, and now over 140,000 knee and hip replacements are performed each year in the UK, revolutionizing the quality of life of patients with painful disabling arthritis.

To be a good orthopaedic surgeon requires not only a wide knowledge base, but also common sense, logic, and practical skills. *A good surgeon knows how to operate; a great surgeon knows when to operate*', is a classic saying that was drilled into me as a young houseman. In this specialty, there are often several management options facing the surgeon and patient, and through careful discussion and the process of informed consent, a joint plan can be formulated and executed.

The questions in this chapter will help you to prepare both for your exams and for a future career as a doctor. ■

TRAUMA AND ORTHOPAEDICS
SINGLE BEST ANSWERS

1. A 17-year-old man is knocked off his moped. He is wearing a helmet and witnesses thought he was travelling at 30mph before impact. Which is the single most appropriate immediate management? ★

A Advanced trauma life support (ATLS) assessment following guidelines

B CT scan of his head

C Glasgow Coma Scale assessment and pupil reaction

D Thorough mechanism of injury history and full examination

E X-rays of chest, pelvis, and cervical spine

2. A motor cyclist has been involved in a motor vehicle collision. He is talking, has bruising on the right side of his chest but normal breath sounds, his pulse rate is 120bpm, and his blood pressure is 60/40mmHg. His Glasgow Coma Scale score is 15/15. He has bruising around his flanks and an obvious open fracture of his right tibia. He has blood at the urethral meatus. His chest X-ray shows some fractured ribs on the right and his pelvic film is shown in Plate 9.1. Which is the single most appropriate next step in his management? ★

A Betadine-soaked dressing, IV antibiotics, and washout of his tibial fracture

B Chest drain for his rib fractures and potential haemothorax

C IV access, IV fluids, and blood replacement

D Pelvic external fixation

E Secure a definitive airway with the anaesthetist

3. A 6-week-old baby with a clicky hip is referred by the health visitor. She has had an ultrasound scan that confirms a dislocated right hip and a dysplastic acetabulum. Which single clinical finding best supports the diagnosis of a dislocated right hip? ★

A Asymmetrical skin creases on the thighs

B Clicking on abduction of the hip

C Dimple at the base of the spine

D Leg length discrepancy

E Limited abduction of the hip on the right

4. An 83-year-old man has had intermittent pain in the base of his spine for 4 months. It has become constant in nature and is not responding to simple analgesics. Which single factor in the history should alert you to the possibility of serious pathology? ★

A Night pain

B Past history of malignancy

C Sciatic pain radiating down the leg from buttock to the foot

D Scoliosis

E Temperature of 38°C or more

5. A 30-year-old woman who is usually fit and well has had intermittent urinary incontinence and loss of sensation around her bottom for the last 24h. Which is the single most appropriate next step in management? ★

A Blood tests, spinal X-rays, and a urine dipstick

B History and examination, including a rectal examination

C Mobilize the theatre team as she needs to go straight to theatre

D Opiate analgesia and senior review

E Urgent MRI scan of the spine

6. A 7-year-old boy has had an intermittent pain in his left hip for the past month. He walks with a slight limp and has decreased abduction at the hip joint. Which is the single most likely diagnosis? ★

A Juvenile idiopathic arthritis

B Missed developmental dysplasia of the hip

C Perthes' disease

D Slipped upper femoral epiphysis

E Transient synovitis

7. A 4-year-old boy has had pain and tenderness in his lower leg for 1 week. He is refusing to weight-bear. There is an area of swelling and warmth at the upper tibia, which is tender. He has a temperature of 39°C. His bloods show:

- White cell count 30 × 10^9/L
- Erythrocyte sedimentation rate (ESR) 110mm/hr
- C-reactive protein (CRP) 200mg/L.

Which is the single most likely causative micro-organism? ★

A *Kingella kingae*

B *Pseudomonas aeruginosa*

C *Salmonella paratyphi*

D *Staphylococcus aureus*

E *Staphylococcus epidermidis*

8. A 70-year-old woman with rheumatoid arthritis is having a total knee replacement. Which is the single most important pre-operative investigation? ★

A Anteroposterior and lateral radiograph of cervical spine

B Dual energy X-ray absorptiometry (DEXA) scanning

C Inflammatory markers

D Chest X-ray

E Up-to-date anteroposterior and lateral X-rays of knee

9. A 6-year-old boy is brought to the Emergency Department with a painful, swollen arm. The mother is unsure what happened and gives a story of an unwitnessed fall off a bunk bed the day before. He has lots of bruising all over his arm and upper body. Which is the single most appropriate management? ★

A Admit the child to the ward and contact your consultant

B Contact the duty social worker

C Discuss your concerns with the paediatrician on call

D Probe the mother about the cause of the bruises

E Send off a full blood count and clotting screen

10. A new born baby has 'clicky' hips at birth. Which single feature is a risk factor for developmental dysplasia of the hip (DDH)? ★

A Family history of DDH

B Low birth weight

C Male sex

D Polyhydramnios

E Second sibling

11. A 45-year-old builder has pins and needles down the medial border of his forearm and weakness in the small muscles in his hand, causing him to drop things. Which is the single name and location of the nerve being compressed? ★

A Anterior interosseous nerve under the fibres of the flexor digitorum sublimis

B Median nerve in the carpal tunnel

C Posterior interosseous nerve under the proximal edge of the supinator

D Ulnar nerve at the cubital tunnel

E Ulnar nerve in Guyon's canal

12. A 65-year-old man sustained a fracture of his femoral neck 4 years ago. He is undergoing a total hip replacement for collapse of the head and secondary osteoarthritis. He walks with a stick, and has an antalgic gait and a significant leg length discrepancy. Which is the single most likely benefit of the procedure? ★

A Equalization of leg length discrepancy

B Improvement of walking distance

C Improvement of range of motion

D Pain relief

E Prevention of compensatory osteoarthritis in other joints

13. A 60-year-old man has a deformed, painless right ankle and foot. He has had blistering and ulceration of his foot in the past. X-rays show a destructive Charcot-type arthropathy of the ankle and subtalar joints. Which is the single most likely underlying diagnosis? ★

A Alcohol-induced peripheral neuropathy

B Diabetes mellitus

C Hereditary motor and sensory neuropathy

D Leprosy

E Tertiary syphillis

14. A 9-year-old boy has put his arm through a glass door. There is significant bleeding from a 5cm deep wound in his forearm. Which is the single most appropriate immediate management? ★

A Apply a high arm tourniquet

B Direct pressure on the axillary artery

C Direct pressure on the wound

D IV antibiotics and tetanus prophylaxis

E Local anaesthetic and clip the bleeding vessel

15. A 25-year-old man has been involved in a drunken brawl and has been knifed in the chest. He is tachypnoeic, tachycardic, hypotensive, and has two stab wounds in the left thorax. Which is the single most appropriate immediate management? ★

A Direct pressure over the stab wounds to stem the bleeding

B Fast bleep the cardiothoracic surgeons

C Get IV access and cross match six units of blood

D Open the airway and give high-flow oxygen

E Open the chest (throacotomy) and begin internal cardiac massage

16. A 7-year-old boy has an open fracture of his forearm. He is on a scout trip away from home and attends with his scout leader. You need to take him to theatre immediately, but cannot get hold of his parents, who are away on holiday. Which is the single most appropriate method of gaining consent for surgery? ★

A Ask a duty social worker to sign the consent form

B Ask another doctor to sign the consent form

C Ask the boy to sign the consent form

D Get the scout leader to sign the consent form

E Written consent is not required as it is an emergency

17. A 75-year-old man attends his 6 week follow-up appointment after a primary right total hip replacement for osteoarthritis. He walks in with the aid of one stick and, as he walks, his upper body sways to the right when he stands on his operated leg. Which is the single best description of his change in gait? ★

A Antalgic

B Normal for this stage in his post-operative recovery

C Short leg

D Trendelenburg positive

E Varus thrust

18. A 36-year-old computer programmer has a painful lump on the volar aspect of his wrist. The lump is well defined, fluctuant, and pulsatile but doesn't transilluminate. Which is the single most appropriate next step in management? ★

A Aspirate the lump in the clinic under local anaesthetic and inject steroid

B Explain the benign nature of the lump and that it is likely to resolve on its own with time

C Organize an ultrasound scan to confirm diagnosis

D Put him on the waiting list for excision under general anaesthetic

E Put him on the waiting list for excision under local anaesthetic

19. A 60-year-old woman has sustained a low-energy fracture of the distal radius. Last year, she fell and sustained a proximal femoral fracture, which was fixed with a dynamic hip screw. A recent DEXA scan has shown a T score of −3. Which is the single most likely diagnosis? ★

A Oligodystrophy

B Osteomalacia

C Osteopenia

D Osteopetrosis

E Osteoporosis

20. A patient is concerned about the risk of deep infection following primary total hip replacement. Which single factor has had the biggest impact on reducing joint replacement infection? ★ ★

A Antibiotic-loaded cement

B Body exhaust suits for the surgeons

C Disposable gowns

D Laminar air flow systems

E Peri-operative prophylactic systemic antibiotics

21. A 60-year-old woman has had neck pain for several years. She now has an acute prolapse of the C5/6 disc, causing nerve root compression on the right side. Which single set of symptoms and signs is she most likely to have? ★ ★

A Dysaesthesia in the thumb and index finger and weakness in elbow extension

B Increased tone and hyper-reflexia in the right arm

C None of these

D Pain and numbness in the medial forearm

E Weakness in elbow flexion and loss of triceps reflex

22. A 2-year-old girl has had multiple bony fractures since birth. She has discoloured teeth, poor growth, and white sclera. Which is the single most likely diagnosis? ★ ★

A Achondroplasia

B Craniocleidodysostosis

C Hypophosphatasia

D Osteogenesis imperfecta

E Osteopetrosis

23. A 50-year-old man has increasing pain in his right knee. His pain is not controlled by daily ibuprofen and paracetamol, and he is particularly troubled going up and down stairs. He has pain even at rest. He had a total meniscectomy 30 years ago after a football injury when he also ruptured his anterior cruciate ligament. His X-ray is shown in Plate 9.2. Which is the single most appropriate management? ★ ★

A Increase his pain medications and get him to use a stick

B Medial unicompartmental knee replacement

C Refer him for physiotherapy

D Steroid injection and review

E Total knee replacement

24. A 25-year-old man has been knocked off his motorcycle. He has an open fracture of his femur. His leg X-ray is shown in Plate 9.3. Which is the single most appropriate definitive management? ★ ★

A External fixator with washout and debridement of the wound and delayed primary closure

B Intramedullary nail with washout and debridement of the wound and delayed primary closure

C Open reduction and plate fixation with washout and debridement of the wound and primary closure

D Washout and debridement of the wound and application of a Thomas splint

E Washout and debridement of the wound and a long leg cast with a window for a vacuum suction pump

25. A baby has been born with a foot deformity, as shown in Plate 9.4. Which is the single best description of this foot deformity? ★ ★

A Calcaneous, abductus, valgus

B Cavus, adductus, varus, equinus

C Cavus, calcaneous, adductus, varus

D Cavus, valgus, equinus

E Pes planus

26. A 20-year-old man falls off his motorbike and fractures his tibial shaft. The management options are discussed with him and he opts for an intramedullary nail. He is put into a backslab cast and listed for surgery the next day. His leg is kept strictly elevated. At 3.30 am, he develops increasing pain despite morphine. Which is the single most appropriate next step in management? ★ ★ ★

A Add a non-steroidal anti-inflammatory drug to his pain relief and review in 30 min

B Call the anaesthetist to set up a morphine patient-controlled analgesia system

C Call your senior; the man needs to go to theatre immediately

D List him for theatre at 6am when his stomach is empty and it is safe to give an anaesthetic

E Split his cast to skin, continue elevation, and review with senior in 15 min

27. A 93-year-old woman is bed-bound in a nursing home and has severe dementia. She has fallen out of bed. Her right hip is stiff but painless, and an X-ray reveals a dislocated total hip replacement (THR). She also has a large 10 × 5cm open pre-tibial laceration. She has a respiratory rate of 23/min with evidence on the ECG of ischaemic changes. Which is the single most appropriate specialty to call to help with the management of this patient? ★ ★ ★

A Anaesthetist to give a general anaesthetic to reduce the THR

B Cardiologist to help interpret the ECG changes

C General medical team to optimize medical care before any intervention

D Plastic surgeon to help manage the open pre-tibial laceration

E Psychiatrist to assess whether she can consent to treatment

28. A 35-year-old man was playing five-a-side football when he thought he had been kicked in the back of the leg. The next day he is hobbling and has pain and swelling around his Achilles tendon. Simmonds' test is equivocal. Which is the single most appropriate investigation to confirm the diagnosis and plan further management? ★ ★ ★ ★

A CT scan

B Examination under anaesthetic

C MRI scan

D Plain X-ray

E Ultrasound scan

29. A 25-year-old man with epilepsy has a painful swollen shoulder after having a fit earlier that day. X-rays are taken, as shown in Plate 9.5. Which is the single most appropriate management? ★ ★ ★ ★

A Organize a CT scan to help plan operative management

B Organize for the patient to go to theatre for a closed reduction

C Organize for the patient to go to theatre for an open reduction

D Reduction using the Hippocratic method under sedation

E Reduction using Kocher's method under sedation

30. A 45-year-old woman has an oblique fracture of her distal fibula. Which is the single best technique to compress the two fragments of bone? ★ ★ ★ ★

A Dynamic compression plate and cancellous screws

B Elastic titanium intramedullary nails

C External fixation with supplementary K-wire fixation

D Lag screw and neutralization plate

E Locking plate with locking screws

31. A 60-year-old man has an acutely painful, swollen knee. 100mL of synovial fluid is aspirated, which is straw-coloured and viscous. Analysis shows no crystals and a white cell count of 4000/mm³ with neutrophils <25%. His pain is much improved after aspiration. Which is the single most likely diagnosis? ★ ★ ★ ★

A Gout

B Pseudogout

C Reactive arthritis

D Rheumatoid arthritis

E Septic arthritis

32. A 45-year-old man has fallen 20 feet off a ladder. As he fell, his right leg got caught in the rungs of the ladder and he felt his knee 'pop in and pop out'. He has a very swollen, tender knee with a cool, white limb and a very faint dorsalis pedis pulse. Which is the single most appropriate immediate management? ★ ★ ★ ★

A Doppler check to assess the pulses more accurately

B MRI of his knee to see which ligaments are damaged

C Mobilize the theatre team immediately; he needs to have an open exploration of the popliteal vessels

D Organize an arteriogram and contact the vascular surgeons for an urgent review

E Organize an urgent fasciotomy to prevent compartment syndrome

33. A 65-year-old man has undergone a primary total hip replacement for osteoarthritis. Post-operatively, he has developed a foot drop, with numbness in his foot and weakness of ankle dorsiflexion to 2/5 power. Which is the single most likely cause of the foot drop? ★ ★ ★ ★

A Axonotmesis of the common peroneal nerve at the head of the fibula due to pressure from positioning during the procedure

B Axonotmesis of the sciatic nerve due to intraoperative traction injury secondary to misplaced retractors

C Neuropraxia of the common peroneal nerve at the head of the fibula due to pressure from positioning during the procedure

D Neuropraxia of the sciatic nerve due to intraoperative traction injury secondary to misplaced retractors

E Neuronotmesis of the sciatic nerve during surgery

34. A 15-year-old boy has fractured his humerus. His X-ray is shown in Plate 9.6. Which is the single most likely mechanism of injury? ★ ★ ★ ★

A Bending force

B Bending force with axial compression

C Direct impact from lateral aspect

D Direct impact from medial aspect

E Torsional force

35. A 13-year-old boy has had repeated ankle sprains, midfoot pain, and problems walking on uneven ground. He has a flat foot that doesn't correct into varus when he stands on tip toes. He also has a stiff subtalar joint. Which is the single most likely diagnosis? ★ ★ ★ ★

A Charcot–Marie–Tooth disease

B Lateral ligament insufficiency (ankle)

C Physiological flexible flat foot

D Sever's disease

E Tarsal coalition

36. A 50-year-old diabetic man has recurrent triggering of the ring finger. The finger is stuck in flexion. It was injected 2 years ago with good results. Which is the single most appropriate management? ★ ★ ★ ★

A Operative release under general anaesthetic

B Operative release under local anaesthetic

C Repeat the injection

D Stretching and a night splint with physiotherapy

E Ultrasound scan to confirm the diagnosis

37. A 22-year-old footballer ruptures his anterior cruciate ligament and tears his medial meniscus after twisting his knee in training. Which single group of clinical findings is most likely 2 weeks after the initial injury? ★ ★ ★ ★

A Effusion, hyperextension, and generalized joint-line tenderness

B Effusion, medial joint-line tenderness, and positive Lachman's test

C Increased opening on valgus stress and tenderness medially

D Increased posterior sag, positive anterior draw, and negative Lachman's test

E Quads wasting, extensor lag, and positive Lachman's test

EXTENDED MATCHING QUESTIONS

Nerve supply of the arm

For each anatomical description, choose the *single* most likely nerve from the list of options below. Each option may be used once, more than once, or not at all. ★

A Anterior interosseous nerve

B Axillary nerve

C Medial cutaneous nerve of forearm

D Median nerve

E Musculocutaneous nerve

F Posterior interosseus nerve

G Radial nerve

H Superficial radial nerve

I Ulnar nerve

1. Found medial to the coracoid process and in close relation to the conjoint tendon; it supplies the biceps brachii and muscles of the anterior compartment of the upper arm.

2. The motor supply of the extensor compartment of the forearm and wrist.

3. At risk from injury on the medial border of the elbow; it supplies the small muscles of the hand.

4. Found in close relation to the humeral head; it can be injured by glenohumeral joint dislocation.

5. Lies in close relation to the humeral diaphysis in the spiral groove; at risk in humeral shaft fractures.

?

Causes of bone tumours

For each patient with a bony tumour, choose the *single* most likely diagnosis from the list of options below. Each option may be used once, more than once, or not at all. ★ ★

A Aneurysmal bone cyst

B Chondrosarcoma

C Chordoma

D Ewing's sarcoma

E Giant cell tumour

F Metastatic lesion

G Osteochondroma

H Osteoid osteoma

I Osteosarcoma

J Soft tissue sarcoma

6. An 80-year-old man has had Paget's disease for 10 years. He now has increasing pain and swelling in his distal femur.

7. A 15-year-old boy has severe night pain in his upper thigh that responds well to aspirin.

8. A 17-year-old woman has pain and local warmth in her lower thigh. An X-ray shows an expansile, lytic lesion and an MRI scan shows that it contains multiple fluid-filled levels.

9. An 80-year-old woman with renal cell carcinoma has a hard fixed breast lump and excruciating lower back pain.

10. A 65-year-old man has had lower back pain, impotence, and tenesmus for several months. He now has acute urinary retention.

Causes of shoulder problems

For each patient with a shoulder problem, choose the *single* most likely diagnosis from the list of options below. Each option may be used once, more than once, or not at all. ★ ★

A Acromioclavicular joint osteoarthritis

B Calcific tendonitis

C Frozen shoulder

D Glenohumeral joint osteoarthritis

E Impingement

F Long head of biceps tendon rupture

G Painful arc syndrome

H Rotator cuff full-thickness tear

I Supraspinatus tendonitis

11. A 30-year-old woman has an acute onset of continuous pain in the shoulder, radiating down the arm. It is so severe that she requires opiate analgesia.

12. An 80-year-old man has global decreased range of motion of the shoulder and night pain.

13. An 65-year-old man has good power in his shoulders but an asymmetrical appearance of the musculature of his upper arms.

14. A 45-year-old woman has a vague story of a bang on the arm. She now has stiffness and inability to sleep on her bad side.

15. A 75-year-old retired farmer has weakness in forward elevation and abduction of his shoulder, although it can be moved passively through the complete range.

Causes of hand and wrist problems

For each patient with pain in the hand, choose the *single* most likely diagnosis from the list of options below. Each option may be used once, more than once, or not at all.

★ ★ ★ ★

A Atypical carpal tunnel

B Carpometacarpal osteoarthritis

C De Quervain's tenosynovitis

D Distal radial fracture

E Flexor carpi radialis tendonitis

F Ganglion

G Intersection syndrome

H Scaphoid fracture

I Scaphotrapeziotrapezium osteoarthritis

J Ulna collateral ligament injury of the thumb

16. A 35-year-old man falls at the dry ski slope on to an outstretched hand. His thumb is swollen and painful to move and there is minimal tenderness at the base of the thumb.

17. A 55-year-old woman has pain at the base of both thumbs. Radiographs show loss of joint space and sclerosis at the joint between the first metacarpal and the trapezium.

18. A 40-year-old woman has tenderness and a soft fullness at the base of the anatomical snuff box of the thumb. There is no history of trauma.

19. A 65-year-old woman falls onto her dominant hand. She has bruising and global tenderness all around the wrist.

20. A 55-year-old woman has had pain at the base of the thumb for a week. Extension against resistance exacerbates the pain, as does palpation over the first dorsal extensor compartment.

Causes of hip and knee problems in children

For each child with pain, choose the *single* most likely diagnosis from the list of options below. Each option may be used once, more than once, or not at all. ★ ★ ★ ★

A Developmental dysplasia of the hip

B Ewing's sarcoma of the pelvis

C Idiopathic coxa vara

D Juvenile idiopathic arthritis

E Perthes' disease

F Septic arthritis

G Slipped upper femoral epiphysis

H Transient synovitis

21. A 7-year-old boy has intermittent pain in his right hip. He is well in himself but has a reduced range of movement, with irritability at the extremes of motion.

22. A 3-year-old girl has a limp. She has a leg length discrepancy of 2cm, shorter on the left, asymmetrical skin creases, and marked limitation in abduction of the left hip.

23. A 13-year-old boy has pain in the groin. Intermittent at first, it is becoming more constant and wakes him up at night. He had a retinoblastoma as a baby.

24. A 6-year-old boy has had intermittent pain, stiffness, and swelling of the knee over the last year. There is an effusion and limitation of flexion.

25. A 12-year-old boy who weighs 75kg has a painful knee and a limp.

Single Best Answers

1. A ★   OHCS 8ᵗʰ edn → p724

Following ATLS guidelines in the *ATLS Handbook* is the appropriate way to treat any significant trauma. The other options may be appropriate further down the line.

2. C ★

In keeping with any significant injury, the immediate priority is to ensure that airway, breathing, and circulation are not compromised. This man's airway and breathing seem secure, so you should move on to treat the potential blood loss from the pelvic fracture by securing circulation.

3. E ★   OHCS 8ᵗʰ edn → p684

Clicking and asymmetry of skin creases are 'soft' signs of hip dislocation. The limitation of abduction suggests a positive Ortolani's test, meaning the hip is out of joint posteriorly.

4. B ★   OHCS 8ᵗʰ edn → p678

This suggests that spinal metastases may be the cause. The other features may also be present with metastatic lesions, but can be features of other diagnoses.

5. B ★   OHCS 8ᵗʰ edn → p676

This history suggests cauda equina syndrome, of which there are many causes. However, the young age makes a sinister cause unlikely. The first step is always a thorough history and examination, and a rectal exam must always be done to assess anal tone.

6. C ★   OHCS 8ᵗʰ edn → p682

In this age group, the most important cause of persistent limp is Perthes' disease, which is an avascular necrosis of the femoral head. Slipped upper femoral epiphysis tends to occur in older, overweight children. Transient synovitis shouldn't last a month. Dysplasia of the hip would have been seen earlier than at 7 years old. Juvenile idiopathic arthritis is possible but less likely.

7. D ★ OHCS 8th edn → p696

This is a picture of osteomyelitis, commonly caused by S. *aureus*.

8. A ★ OHCS 8th edn → p613–614

There are guidelines in most hospitals about which pre-operative investigations to perform. However, patients with rheumatoid arthritis are at risk of cervical involvement, which can make anaesthetic management difficult. If in doubt, always discuss with an anaesthetist.

9. C ★ OHCS 8th edn → p146

Any doctor who sees children needs to be aware of possible non-accidental injury. However, whilst it is important to document exactly what you found, there will be a doctor for child protection, either a paediatric middle grade or a consultant, who can seek further information and plan appropriate management.
→ http://www.everychildmatters.gov.uk/socialcare/safeguarding/workingtogether/

10. A ★ OHCS 8th edn → p684

The risk factors for DDH are:
Female
First born
Foot first (breech)
Family history
Further bony abnormalities, e.g. talipes equinovarus

11. D ★ OHCS 8th edn → p666

12. D ★ OHCS 8th edn → p706

The main benefit of hip replacement is pain control. Improvement in mobility is much less successful.

13. B ★

His age makes hereditary motor and sensory neuropathy unlikely. Diabetes is the commonest cause of neuropathy, leading to arthropathy.

14. C ★

Following ABC (airway, breathing, and circulation) guidelines, the first step in controlling bleeding is direct pressure. Once this is under control, he may need further surgical intervention, and antibiotics and tetanus prophylaxis may be indicated, but these are not the priorities.

15. D ★

Following advanced trauma life support (ATLS) guidance, securing an airway always comes before anything else.

16. E ★

Only a person with parental responsibility can give valid consent on behalf of a child who is not Gillick competent. In some cases, the parent may sign over parental responsibility to another adult, but usually this does not happen. In an emergency, the doctor should document the need for an emergency procedure clearly and why it is needed, but can proceed to save life or limb without formal written consent.

→ http://www.gmc-uk.org/guidance/ethical_guidance/consent_guidance/Consent_guidance.pdf

17. D ★   OHCS 8th edn → p680

The Trendelenburg test tests the stability of the hip. When the patient stands on the affected leg, the pelvis falls on the opposite side, causing the upper body to lurch to the affected side to compensate. This is a positive test. It is caused by weak abductor muscles, a dislocated hip, or the absence of a stable fulcrum.

18. C ★   OHCS 8th edn → p668

This is the classic location and description of a ganglion – a benign bulge of synovium. It may resolve spontaneously, but, if painful, can be aspirated or excised. However, diagnosis should be confirmed first with soft-tissue imaging.

19. E ★

DEXA stands for dual-energy X-ray absorptiometry and is considered the most accurate test for bone density. Whilst standard X-rays show changes in bone density after about 40% bone loss, a DEXA scan can detect changes after about a 1% change. The results of a DEXA scan are reported in two ways: as T scores and as Z scores. A T score compares bone density with the optimal peak bone density for gender. It is reported as the number of standard deviations below the mean. A T score of greater than −1 is considered normal. A T score of −1 to −2.5 is considered to be osteopenia and at risk of developing osteoporosis. A T score of less than −2.5 is diagnostic of osteoporosis.

20. E ★★

21. A ★★   OHCS 8ᵗʰ edn → pp660, 716–7, 762–3

Knowledge of the specific patterns of nerve damage are useful in diagnosis. See the tables and pictures in OHCS.

22. D ★★

These are the features of some types of osteogenesis imperfecta, a rare cause of multiple fractures. These signs may help suspicion of the diagnosis.

23. E ★★   OHCS 8ᵗʰ edn → p706

This man has exhausted non-operative measures for management of his osteoarthritis and warrants surgical treatment. His X-ray shows medial compartment osteoarthritis. However, he requires a total knee replacement because a unicompartmental knee replacement is contraindicated in a patient without an anterior cruciate ligament.

24. B ★★   OHCS 8ᵗʰ edn → p752

Intramedullary nails align and stabilize the bone and share the load with the bone. They allow early mobilization. Because the fracture is open, it needs careful washing out. Delayed primary closure refers to the initial debridement and then closing of the wound at a later stage. This allows better healing of contaminated wounds.

25. B ★★   OHCS 8ᵗʰ edn → p684

This is an image of club foot, or talipes equinovarus. A full club foot involves the ankle (talus) and foot (pes), and is equinus (the heel is elevated like a horse's) and cavus (with an exaggerated arch). It is varus (turned inward) and adducted (moved towards the midline). It cannot be moved through the normal range of movements and the Achilles is tight and the calf muscle shortened..

26. E ★★★   OHCS 8ᵗʰ edn → p734

Leg fractures run the risk of development of compartment syndrome, inflammation, and swelling within a closed fascial compartment, leading to impaired blood supply. However, this man is in a cast, so simple relief of the external pressure and elevation may alleviate the pain and swelling. If the pain continues, he may be developing compartment syndrome and need fasciotomy, so a close review is essential.

27. C ★★★

This situation is not uncommon. The patient is more likely to suffer harm as a result of their medical illness than with their dislocated THR, and medical problems should be co-managed with medical teams in the interest of best patient outcome.

28. E ★ ★ ★ ★ OHCS 8ᵗʰ edn → p712

A ruptured Achilles tendon causes sudden pain when running or jumping and the heel cannot be raised from the floor when standing on the affected leg. In Simmonds' test, the patient kneels on a chair and the calf is squeezed; there will be less plantar flexion of the foot on the affected side. An ultrasound scan is the easiest and most discriminatory test for soft tissue injuries, although it is operator dependent.

29. A ★ ★ ★ ★ OHCS 8ᵗʰ edn → p740

The radiographs show a locked posterior dislocation of the glenohumeral joint. This is often a missed injury as the signs (positive 'light bulb' sign) are subtle on the anterioposterior view. The diagnosis is obvious on the axillary view. This is a difficult problem and often further imaging is necessary to plan surgical management.

30. D ★ ★ ★ ★ OHCS 8ᵗʰ edn → p754

A lag screw is the best technique to produce interfragmentary compression in the context of absolute stability. This allows the fracture to heal by primary bone healing without the formation of a callus.

31. C ★ ★ ★ ★ OHCS 8ᵗʰ edn → pp708–709

Analysis of colour, viscosity, and composition of synovial fluid is important. Here, the straw colour and high viscosity but low number of neutrophils point to a non-inflammatory cause. In inflammation or infection, the fluid is yellow with a high number of neutrophils.

32. D ★ ★ ★ ★

The history and examination findings alert you to a possible knee dislocation that has self-reduced. This comes with a significant risk to the neurovascular bundle. An arteriogram is the gold standard investigation with an urgent review by the vascular surgeons.

33. D ★ ★ ★ ★

Neuropraxia (physiological conduction block) is the most common type of nerve injury encountered usually due to compression on the nerve. In total hip replacement, misplaced retractors are the usual cause for this, and the sciatic nerve is the most common nerve involved.

34. E ★ ★ ★ ★

This is a spiral fracture, which is caused by a twisting force.

35. E ★ ★ ★ ★

Tarsal coalition – an abnormal connection between the tarsal bones – commonly presents in adolescence as the connection ossifies as the child grows. Often, there is a history of repeated ankle sprains and difficulty walking on uneven ground.

36. B ★ ★ ★ ★ OHCS 8th edn → p668

Diabetics are renowned for having recurrent resistant triggering digits. Operative release under local anaesthetic avoids the complications of a general anaesthetic (which are increased in a diabetic) and allows the surgeon to check the release by asking the patient to move the finger intraoperatively.

37. B ★ ★ ★ ★ OHCS 8th edn → p686

He is likely to have a residual effusion at 2 weeks after a significant knee injury. Joint-line tenderness is a non-specific examination finding in a knee with intra-articular damage. Lachman's test, performed with the knee in 30° of flexion, is the most sensitive clinical test to diagnose an anterior cruciate ligament injury. Important points are to compare with the other knee and the presence or absence of an end point.

Extended Matching Questions

1. E ★
2. F ★
3. I ★
4. B ★
5. G ★

General feedback on 1–5: OHCS 8th edn → p762

→ http://www.instantanatomy.net/arm/nerves/general.html
→ http://www.surgical-tutor.org.uk/default-home.htm

6. I ★ ★
7. H ★ ★
8. A ★ ★
9. F ★ ★
10. C ★ ★

General feedback on 6–10: OHCS 8th edn → p698. Bone tumours can be benign or malignant. Most malignant bone tumours are metastases from distant primaries. Even benign bone tumours can cause pain, swelling, and fractures.

Osteosarcoma is the commonest primary bone malignancy and typically occurs in growing areas of bone. Although it is most frequently found in teenagers, Paget's disease, the increased production of new bone, is a risk factor. In this case, the pain and swelling would increase. Ewing's sarcoma is also a primary malignant tumour that typically occurs in the pelvis and long bones in teenagers. Chondrosarcomas arise from cartilage and occur in the axial skeleton of middle-aged people and present with a lump. Giant cell tumour is an osteolytic lesion that again typically occurs around epiphyses of young adults. Metastases tend to go to the spine, ribs, and pelvis. Breast, prostate, lung, kidney, and colon carcinomas all spread to bone. Chordoma is a rare, slow-growing bone malignancy that develops in remnants of the embryonic notochord. It typically occurs at the base of the spine or skull and causes compression of the spinal cord.

Benign tumours include osteochondroma, which is a cartilaginous overgrowth that causes a painless lump. Osteoid osteoma presents as a painful area, often in the tibia or femur, and often causing night pain relieved by non-steroidal anti-inflammatory drugs.

An aneursymal bone cyst is an expansile, osteolytic lesion that may arise in tumours or following a bone injury. They can arise in any bone and typically cause fairly quick development of pain and local swelling with local skin warmth and restricted joint movement. They look cystic on imaging.

11. B ★★

This is a build up of calcium in the rotator cuff tendons, which is acutely painful and probably one of the most painful conditions in the shoulder. It can also cause impingement when lifting the arm.

12. D ★★

Shoulder osteoarthritis is less common than in other joints, but risk increases with age or previous injury. The pain and stiffness is progressive and limits movement in all directions.

13. F ★★

This feels like something going when it happens and causes a golf-ball-like swelling in the biceps on flexion of the elbow.

14. C ★★

A frozen shoulder describes a condition where the shoulder is almost completely immovable due to inflammation of the capsule and ligaments. It may be triggered by injury. There is a phase of pain and progressive loss of motion, and then resolution of the pain with worsening stiffness that may take a couple of years to resolve.

15. H ★★

Specific limitation of movement leads to the relevant anatomy. Shoulder movement is complex and controlled by several muscles, which come into play at different points in movement. Tears in tendons in the rotator cuff limit active movement.

General feedback on 11–15: OHCS 8th edn → pp662–664

→ http://www.shoulderdoc.co.uk/

16. J ★★★★

The ulna collateral ligament is typically injured by a fall onto a hand with the thumb out, causing it to bend back. It causes pain and swelling at the base of the thumb, where the metacarpophalangeal joint is. It is also called gamekeeper's thumb.

17. B ★★★★

Osteoarthritis is common, and typical findings are loss of joint space and sclerosis on X-ray.

18. F ★★★★

A ganglion is a soft-tissue, benign swelling that occurs on or around the joints or tendons in the hand and foot.

19. D ★★★★

Falls onto outstretched hands can damage anywhere along the arm from the thumb to the shoulder, depending on factors such as age and the mechanism of injury. The location of swelling, pain, and bruising indicates the area of damage. In post-menopausal women, wrist fractures are common after falls.

20. C ★★★★

This is inflammation of the tendons at the base of the thumb. It causes localized pain and swelling. Finkelstein's manoeuvre is worsening of pain when the thumb is folded across the palm and the fingers folded over the top.

General feedback on 16–20: OHCS 8th edn → pp742–746

→ http://www.handuniversity.com/

21. E ★★★★

This osteochondritis of the femoral head presents in children aged 3–11 years and in boys more often than girls. It causes limitation of movement in all directions.

22. A ★ ★ ★ ★

Despite neonatal screening, dislocated hips are still missed. In this case, children may walk late or with a limp.

23. B ★ ★ ★ ★

Pain that wakes someone at night should always be taken seriously. In this case, the past history of a malignancy should raise concern about another malignancy. Ewing's sarcoma usually presents in adolescence.

24. D ★ ★ ★ ★

The story of recurrent pain and swelling suggests a chronic condition. Juvenile idiopathic arthritis is an inflammatory arthritis so will cause effusion, warmth, and limited movement.

25. G ★ ★ ★ ★

This occurs in peripubertal, overweight children, boys more often than girls. It causes limp and pain in the groin or knee, although these may be mild.

General feedback on 20-25: OHCS 8th edn →pp682, 684, 698

CHAPTER 10

EMERGENCY MEDICINE

Ruth Brown

Emergency medicine is not all 'ER', glamour, and fast-moving action. Much of it requires caring for relatively minor problems or complex elderly patients. A solid knowledge of basic sciences is essential to support the clinical and practical management decisions, and you need to know the acute presentations of all specialties. This requires a lot of study as well as a sensible approach to finding information on unknown conditions while you are working. No one can know everything, but having a system to approach a problem and applying basic principles helps.

Gathering information rapidly is important. Gaining clues from the patient and their relative is useful, as is information on events at the scene from the ambulance paramedics. Hospital notes are often not available and neither is the GP, so you have to make decisions on limited information. Rather than making definitive diagnoses confirmed by expensive tests, the role of the emergency physician is to determine the immediate threat to life or limb and treat that threat, while gathering information to make a 'most likely' diagnosis so that treatment can start. Observing the patient in a clinical decision unit can often help to confirm your suspicions, give you further information on how severe a condition is, or eliminate a possible diagnosis.

Ultimately, emergency medicine requires assessing risk, evaluating the added benefit of admission over discharge, and excellent communication. The only way to learn emergency medicine is to practise, discuss patients, and develop your analytical and decision-making skills. These questions are designed to develop some of those skills, showing you an approach to solving the clinical problems commonly encountered in the Emergency Department, how to use tests efficiently and effectively, and some of the options for treatment that are available other than admission under inpatient teams. ∎

EMERGENCY MEDICINE
SINGLE BEST ANSWERS

1. A 24-year-old man is hit by a car travelling at 50mph. He is unconscious at the scene and there are only two rescuers. He has an obvious fracture of his right leg and swelling of his abdomen. Which is the single most appropriate immediate management of this patient's assumed cervical spine injury at the scene? ★

A Collar, sand bags, and tape

B Halo traction

C Manual in-line immobilization

D Manual in-line traction

E Soft sponge collar

2. A 56-year-old man has had chest pain for 3h. The pain came on suddenly when he arrived at a London hotel after travelling from Scotland by train. The pain is sharp and worse on breathing. He is a smoker. Which single investigation will be the most useful to confirm the likely diagnosis? ★

A Arterial blood gas

B Chest X-ray

C D-dimer

D Immediate troponin

E Serial ECGs

3. A 46-year-old woman is in a coma. Her partner tells you that she has had abdominal pain and vomiting for 3 days. She is clinically dehydrated. Her blood sugar is 48mmol/L and her arterial pH is 7.0. Which is the single most appropriate immediate management? ★

A Bolus of normal saline

B Cefuroxime and metronidazole IV

C Insulin infusion of short-acting insulin at 10U/h

D Normal saline 2L with potassium 40mmol/L over 4h

E Prochlorperazine IV

4. A 45-year-old man has a 2cm laceration to the radial border of the middle and distal phalanx of his right index finger. Which is the single most appropriate local anaesthetic to use to close the wound? ★

A 0.5% bupivocaine without epinephrine (adrenaline)

B 1% lidocaine with epinephrine (adrenaline) 1:1000

C 1% lidocaine without epinephrine (adrenaline)

D 2% lidocaine with epinephrine (adrenaline) 1:1000

E 5% prilocaine without epinephrine (adrenaline)

5. A 40-year-old woman has pain and discharge from her right ear, a temperature of 38.3°C, a blocked nose, and a mild cough. She had a slight pain and deafness in her right ear 1 week ago, which she treated with warm olive oil dripped into her ear. She is a telebanking operator who uses a head set with an ear piece in her right ear. Which is the single most likely diagnosis? ★

A Extensive wax in the ear

B Foreign body in the ear

C Otitis externa

D Otitis media

E Perforated ear drum

6. A 56-year-old man has had a fall. He has a fracture of the radial head, which is undisplaced. Which is the single most appropriate method of immobilizing this fracture? ★

A Above-arm backslab

B Broad arm sling

C Collar and cuff

D Futura splint

E High arm sling

7. An 85-year-old man has an epistaxis. He is on warfarin for atrial fibrillation. Which single drug that he has been recently started on is most likely to be related to the cause of the epistaxis? ★

A Aspirin

B Bendroflumethiazide

C Clopidogrel

D Erythromycin

E Penicillin

8. An 89-year-old woman has had multiple falls. She has been to the Emergency Department 30 times in the last 6 months but has only been admitted once. You assess her and can find little acutely wrong with her, but are concerned about sending her home. She appears to be unsteady on her feet. Which single service would be most helpful in contributing to a management plan? ★

A GP

B Hospital chiropody

C Hospital optician

D Medical registrar

E Occupational therapy

9. A 72-year-old man is brought to the Emergency Department in shock. His systolic blood pressure is 76mmHg, with a pulse rate of 120 beats/min. He has a history of bleeding from ulcers in his stomach and has melaena on rectal examination. Which is the single most appropriate immediate management? ★

A Application of a MAST (military antishock trousers) suit

B IV bolus of gelofusin

C IV bolus of 5% dextrose

D IV infusion of noradrenaline (norepinephrine)

E Transfusion of packed red blood cells

10. A 27-year-old man has a sudden onset of a severe occipital headache. Which single clinical sign is of greatest concern? ★

A Loss of consciousness

B Neck stiffness

C Photophobia

D Unilateral pain

E Vomiting

11. A 45-year-old man has a systolic blood pressure of 50mmHg and a pulse rate of 120 beats/min. Which single vascular access lines would be the best to use? ★

A Green venflon (18G)

B Grey venflon (16G)

C Intraosseus needle

D Single-lumen central line

E Triple-lumen central line

12. A 45-year-old scaffolder has fallen 30 feet from the scaffold. He is unconscious and brought in on a spinal board. You wish to 'log roll' him off the spinal board. Which single instruction to the team about a log roll should be given? ★

A A rectal examination must be performed first

B Five members of staff are required in total

C One staff member takes the shoulders and pelvis

D The head must be held slightly flexed on the body

E The staff member who examines the back is in charge

13. A 23-year-old woman has been tackled during a football match and has a fracture of the tibial plateau, which is undisplaced. Which is the single most appropriate method of immobilizing this fracture? ★

A Above-knee backslab

B Below-knee backslab

C Cast brace

D Cricket bat splint

E Wool and crepe bandage

14. A 2-year-old boy is brought to the Emergency Department from his nursery. They are concerned because he has multiple bruises on his arms and legs. Which single injury is the most likely to be non-accidental? ★

A Bruising to the anterior shins

B Dislocation of the radial head

C Greenstick fracture of the distal radius

D Hot water splash burns to the arm and face

E Small, round bruises to the sides of the chest

15. A 75-year-old man has an acutely red left eye and is vomiting. His visual acuity is 6/24 and he appears very unwell. The eye is red and the cornea hazy, and the pupil is irregular and unreactive. Which is the single most likely diagnosis? ★

A Acute closed angle glaucoma

B Central retinal vein thrombosis

C Conjunctivitis

D Episcleritis

E Herpetic ulcer

16. A 34-year-old man is crushed against a wall by a reversing car. He is distressed and has difficulty breathing. Which is the single most reliable sign of a right-sided tension pneumothorax? ★

A Absent breath sounds on the right side

B Dullness of the chest to percussion

C Hyper-resonance to percussion

D The presence of circulatory shock

E Tracheal deviation to the left

17. A 25-year-old man has had a generalized seizure lasting 5min. He remains post-ictal and his breathing is noisy. Which single piece of equipment is the most appropriate to use to maintain a patent airway? ★

A Endotracheal tube

B Guedel airway

C Nasopharyngeal airway

D Suction

E Tracheostomy tube

18. A 6-week-old boy has been vomiting immediately after every feed for the last 5 days. He vomits large quantities of non-bilious vomitus, which shoot out all over his mother while she feeds him. He is screaming hungrily and has sunken eyes and dry mucous membranes. Which is the single most likely diagnosis? ★

A Hirschsprung's disease

B Malrotation of the bowel

C Oesophageal atresia

D Pyloric stenosis

E Urinary tract infection

19. A 54-year-old railway worker is hit by a train. He has an open injury to his right thigh with a fractured femur clearly visible in the wound. There is arterial bleeding from the wound and his systolic blood pressure is 70mmHg. Which is the single most appropriate immediate action? ★

A Activate the major haemorrhage protocol

B Apply a tourniquet proximally

C Apply pressure to the wound

D Ask the surgeon to cross-clamp the femoral artery

E Explore the wound to clamp the bleeding vessel

20. A 35-year-old man has acute pain in his upper abdomen radiating through to his back and is vomiting. Which single factor is most likely to support a diagnosis of pancreatitis? ★

A Contact with gastroenteritis

B Excessive alcohol intake

C History of foreign travel

D History of renal colic

E Use of cocaine and amphetamines

21. A 25-year-old woman has vaginal bleeding. Her husband tells you that they have been undergoing fertility treatment and she is thought to be 2 months pregnant after implantation of fertilized eggs. She has some bleeding from her vagina with mild left-sided abdominal tenderness. She has a pulse rate of 70 beats/min and a systolic blood pressure of 80mmHg. Which is the single most appropriate action to take in the Emergency Department? ★

A Arrange an urgent ultrasound scan of her pelvis

B Arrange for her to go to theatre

C Give her O-negative blood

D Give her O-positive blood

E Perform a speculum examination

22. A 45-year-old man presents with tachycardia and the ECG shown in Plate 10.1. Which single feature is thought to be an adverse sign in patients with this condition? ★ ★

A Abdominal pain

B Agitation and confusion

C Systolic blood pressure over 180mmHg

D Redness of the extremities

E Basal crepitations and raised jugular venous pressure

23. A 25-year-old woman has taken 40 paracetamol tablets (20g). She is refusing to accept medical treatment, stating that she wishes to die. Which is the single most appropriate immediate course of action? ★ ★

A Allow her to go home as everyone has a right to die

B Assume she is mentally incompetent and treat her against her wishes

C Contact her GP for more information about her

D Formally assess her capacity to refuse treatment

E Request psychiatry to section her for medical treatment

24. A 95-year-old woman has a leg ulcer on the medial aspect of her lower leg. It is weeping, with necrotic tissue in the centre of the ulcer. After debridement under local anaesthetic, the wound looks pink and has some minor bleeding areas. Which is the single most appropriate dressing to apply? ★ ★

A Alginate dressing

B Flamazine cream

C Iodine-impregnated dressing

D Jelonet® dressing

E Non-adherent dressing

25. A 43-year-old woman is in a coma. Her eyes open to pain, she responds with groans to pain, and she extends to pain. Which is her single Glasgow Coma Scale score? ★

A 3

B 6

C 9

D 12

E 15

26. A 68-year-old man is pronounced dead in the department after a prolonged resuscitation. Which single factor in the history requires reporting of the death to the coroner/procurator fiscal? ★ ★ ★

A The death is related to a diagnosed terminal illness

B The death is related to an industrial disease

C The death is related to travel overseas

D The patient had seen his GP in the last 2 days

E The patient is not a UK citizen

27. You are walking home from work as a foundation doctor near the railway line when you hear a massive noise. A mainline train has derailed and is on its side. There appear to be multiple casualties. Which is the single most appropriate action? ★ ★ ★

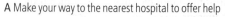

A Make your way to the nearest hospital to offer help

B Provide immediate first aid to the nearest casualty

C Telephone 999 and give a formal report

D Telephone the press to give them the news

E Telephone your hospital to let them know

28. An 18-year-old man has been fitting for the last 15min. An oxygen mask is in place and a nasal airway has been inserted by the ambulance crew. One dose of rectal diazepam has been given and a cannula has been inserted. Which is the single most appropriate immediate treatment? ★ ★ ★

A Diazepam 10mg per rectum

B Lorazepam 4mg IV

C Midazolam 4mg IV

D Phenytoin 18mg/kg IV

E Thiopentone 5mg/kg IV

29. A 75-year-old diabetic woman has a pre-tibial laceration to her right leg that she sustained 45min ago. She has a barely palpable popliteal pulse and no pulses in the foot. Which is the single most appropriate method of closure? ★ ★ ★ ★

A 30 Ethibond (semi-synthetic) sutures

B 40 Vicryl Rapide sutures

C Primary skin grafting

D Steristrips

E Tissue glue

30. A 72-year-old man is acutely short of breath and unwell, his oxygen saturation on air is 75% and his blood gases show a mildly raised carbon dioxide and a low oxygen level with a mild mixed acidosis. Which single factor is a contraindication to the use of non-invasive ventilation in this patient? ★ ★ ★ ★

A Epistaxis

B False teeth

C Nausea

D Pneumonia

E Previous respiratory arrest

31. A 75-year-old man has collapsed. He has left-sided facial weakness and a dense left hemiparesis. He is looking towards his right side and appears to have left-sided neglect. There is no obvious visual-field deficit. He has severe dysarthria but no obvious dysphasia. The CT brain scan performed at 6h is suggestive of an ischaemic area in the distribution of the right middle cerebral artery. Which single intervention is most likely to optimize his outcome? ★ ★ ★ ★

A Control his heart rate to between 60 and 100 beats/min

B Control his temperature above 37.5°C

C Keep his systolic blood pressure below 100mmHg

D Maintain his blood glucose within normal range

E Maintain his haemoglobin above 12g/dL

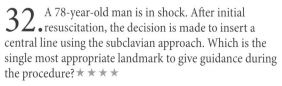

32. A 78-year-old man is in shock. After initial resuscitation, the decision is made to insert a central line using the subclavian approach. Which is the single most appropriate landmark to give guidance during the procedure? ★ ★ ★ ★

A Insertion is at the junction of the medial and middle thirds of the clavicle

B The clavicle is superior to the subclavian vein

C The needle should be pointing towards the tip of the contralateral scapula

D The subclavian vein lies medial to the subclavian artery

E The subclavian vein runs under the first rib

33. You are asked to act as team leader in the resuscitation of a 30-year-old man. Which is the single most effective behaviour of a team leader? ★ ★ ★ ★

A Check all team members' identity and skills when they arrive

B Continually ask team members their opinion

C Insist on silence during the resuscitation unless asked directly

D Issue all instructions in a loud voice

E Personally perform all invasive procedures

EXTENDED MATCHING QUESTIONS

Causes of chest pain

For each patient with chest pain, choose the *single* most likely diagnosis from the list of options below. Each option may be used once, more than once, or not at all. ★

A Acute coronary syndrome

B Costochondritis

C Myocardial infarction

D Pneumonia

E Pulmonary embolism

F Reflux oesophagitis

G Shingles

H Tuberculosis

1. A 25-year-old woman has had a sharp left-sided chest pain for 4h. She fractured her ankle 4 weeks ago falling down some stairs on her way outside for a cigarette and has been in a plaster cast.

2. A 65-year-old man has had central crushing chest pain and palpitations for 2h. An ECG shows new left-bundle branch block.

3. A 54-year-old woman has an area on her right chest wall that is excruciatingly painful to touch. There is some redness in a linear distribution over the tender area.

4. A 45-year-old woman has central crushing pain in her chest that wakes her at night and improves on sitting up.

5. A 35-year-old man who is human immunodeficiency virus (HIV)-positive has had right-sided pleuritic chest pain and a productive cough with green sputum for 2 days.

Use of airway adjuncts

For each presentation, choose the *single* most appropriate airway adjunct required from the list of options below. Each option may be used once, more than once, or not at all. ★

A Bag valve mask

B Endotracheal tube

C Guedel airway

D High-flow oxygen with a reservoir mask

E Nasopharyngeal airway

F Surgical airway

G Tracheostomy

H Venturi mask with 24% oxygen

6. A 25-year-old man is recovering from a grand mal seizure, which lasted 6min and was terminated by a single dose of diazepam.

7. An 85-year-old man with chronic obstructive pulmonary disease (COPD) has a respiratory tract infection and a respiratory rate of 25/min.

8. A 56-year-old man has had a serious head and facial injury and his Glasgow Coma Scale score is 6/15.

9. A 45-year-old woman has been in a house fire and has severe burns around the face, soot in the mouth, stridor, and singed eyebrows.

10. A 10-year-old boy with severe asthma is unable to talk in sentences.

Acute pain relief

For each presentation, choose the *single* most appropriate method of immediate pain relief from the list of options below. Each option may be used once, more than once, or not at all. ★ ★

A Diclofenac 75mg IM

B Dispersible paracetamol 1g oral

C Glyceryl trinitrate 1 spray sublingual

D Immediate reduction

E Immobilization with a splint

F Inhaled nitrous oxide

G Morphine 2–10mg titrated IV

H Oramorph 0.5mg/kg oral

11. A 56-year-old man has had acute central chest pain for 5min. He is a smoker and has a strong family history of ischaemic heart disease.

12. A 36-year-old man falls from his bicycle and has a dislocated right shoulder. He is in pain and there is a lot of muscle spasm around the shoulder.

13. A 4-year-old boy slips and dislocates his right little finger proximal interphalangeal joint.

14. A 25-year-old woman has a high temperature and very painful swollen tonsils.

15. A 35-year-old man has severe right-sided abdominal and loin pain, colicky in nature, which radiates to his right testis.

Immobilization of fractures

For each presentation, choose the *single* most appropriate method of immobilization from the list of options below. Each option may be used once, more than once, or not at all. ★ ★ ★

A Broad arm sling

B Collar and cuff

C Colles' plaster

D Futura splint

E High arm sling

F Mallet finger splint

G Neighbour strapping

H Scaphoid plaster

16. A 25-year-old man who has had an anterior dislocation of his shoulder reduced under IV sedation.

17. An 85-year-old man with a minimally displaced fracture of the surgical neck of his right humerus.

18. A 45-year-old man with pain and crepitus over Lister's tubercle of the right radius, with a normal X-ray.

19. A 25-year-old man with a boxer's fracture of the right fifth metacarpal.

20. A 43-year-old woman with an infected dog bite to the distal phalanx of the left index finger.

EMERGENCY MEDICINE ANSWERS

Single Best Answers

1. A ★   OHCS 8th edn → p798

In any major trauma, cervical spine protection is considered along with the airway. Full protection entails a rigid collar correctly sized and immobilization with sandbags and tape. Manual in-line immobilization should be used until these are available.

2. C ★

This man has risk factors for a pulmonary embolus (smoking and travel) and the history is suspicious of this. Whilst many of these investigations should be performed in suspected pulmonary embolus, the D-dimer result, if positive, indicates the diagnosis. However, if negative in a patient with a good history, then clinical suspicion should still be high.

3. A ★

This woman has a markedly raised blood sugar and is acidotic, indicating diabetic ketoacidosis. After control of airway and breathing, which should always come first, the priority is to restore circulating volume with a fluid bolus.

4. C ★   OHCS 8th edn → p632

1–2mL of 1% lidocaine is sufficient for the majority of wounds. Ring blocks essentially use infiltration of local anaesthetic into the soft tissue around the digital nerve, resulting in nerve impulses being blocked before they reach the spinal cord and the cerebral cortex, thus achieving anaesthesia. Two injections are required, one on each side of the finger at the base of the finger. The whole skin of the finger will be anaesthetized by such a block, including the nail bed. 2% lidocaine does not confer any great value over 1% and Emergency Departments are recommended to keep only one strength to minimize the risk of confusion when calculating doses. Using adrenaline (epinephrine) in any local infiltration around an end artery (the digital artery) is contraindicated because of the risk to perfusion to the distal finger. Other end arteries include the nasal artery and the artery to the penis.

5. D ★   OHCS 8th edn → p544

She is most likely to have developed otitis media in association with her viral upper respiratory tract infection, which has led to a perforation of her drum and discharge of the pus. It is unlikely that her symptoms are from a simple otitis externa, as this rarely gives systemic symptoms such as fever in an adult. Although a foreign body may act as a nidus for infection, it is unlikely that her ear piece has migrated into her ear without being noticed. Wax should not cause systemic upset. An isolated perforation of the ear drum should not cause continued discharge or temperature.

6. B ★   OHCS 8th edn → p740

The objective of the immobilization must be considered: this fracture will heal well in time and there are no strong forces working across the fracture site to displace the fracture. Therefore the key aim of the immobilization is pain relief. A broad arm sling is the most comfortable method of immobilizing the arm, as it allows support for the whole arm and supports the elbow itself. A high arm sling flexes the elbow to over 90° and therefore is uncomfortable in the presence of an elbow effusion. A collar and cuff is used by some authorities, but confers no advantage and allows the elbow to feel the full effects of gravity, which some patients find uncomfortable. A Futura splint (a removable splint that immobilizes the wrist) is not appropriate for the elbow. A backslab is difficult to apply and when strong enough to keep the elbow from moving will be very heavy. It is not necessary to completely immobilize the joint in this patient.

7. D ★

Erythromycin can inhibit the metabolism of warfarin by affecting the cytochrome P450 complex in the liver and therefore enhance its effects.

8. E ★

This is quite common in the elderly and consideration should be given to making sure it does not keep happening. Occupational therapy services can assess the home environment and daily functioning, and can address issues that may predispose to falls.

9. B ★   OHCS 8th edn → p726

The priority is fluid resuscitation of the circulating volume. There is an ongoing debate about the use of crystalloid versus colloid solution

for this. However, dextrose would not be an appropriate choice
of crystalloid solution. Blood would not be given as the primary
resuscitation fluid, but may be needed later in significant bleeding.

10. A ★

The sudden onset of severe occipital headache suggests a
subarachnoid haemorrhage. All of these symptoms may occur in a
patient with a subarachnoid haemorrhage, but loss of consciousness
suggests rising intracranial pressure and is an emergency.

11. B ★

This man is significantly shocked and needs fluid resuscitation. A large-
bore line is needed, but central lines take too long to insert. Intraosseus
needles may be appropriate in young children, but vascular access
should be possible in adults.

12. B ★   OHCS 8ᵗʰ edn → p774

A log roll is performed with five people: one stands at the head and
keeps control of the head, neck and airway and gives commands; one
takes the arms and trunk; one takes the upper legs and pelvis; one
supports the calves; and the fifth examines the back and performs
a rectal examination. The patient is rolled gently towards the 3
supporters of the body and kept held in a stable line while the back is
examined.

13. A ★   OHCS 8ᵗʰ edn → p754

The most important issue in this fracture is to consider what is attached
to the fracture site and therefore what the possible displacement or
consequences of not immobilizing might be. The tibial plateau is a
weight-bearing surface and so any fracture must be treated as non-
weight bearing at first. In addition, the injury pattern often includes
injuries to the menisci or collateral ligaments. If the fracture involves
the cruciate ligaments (evidenced by involvement of the tibial spine in
the fracture line), then minimizing the anterioposterior movement of
the tibia on the femur is important.

Immobilization techniques must be easy for the patient to manage,
and maintain their mobility. Therefore, the most appropriate technique
for immobilization in the Emergency Department is the above-knee
backslab. A below-knee backslab will not restrict the anterioposterior
movement of the tibia on the femur. The cast brace is more suitable
once the patient has started to mobilize the knee after the initial
injury has settled. A cricket bat splint may be useful as it will allow the
patient to wash their leg but may not be available in the Emergency
Department. A wool and crepe bandage was a useful method but is

no longer used because of the extensive resources required and the difficulty for the patient in keeping such a bandage correctly applied.

14. E ★   OHCS 8th edn → p146

Accidents are common in toddlers and the difficulty can be working out which are non-accidental. The shins are a very common site for bruising, but the chest, abdomen, and back are not. Small, discrete, round bruises are suggestive of fingers or an implement. Pulled elbows and greenstick fractures are common in young children, and burns that have splash patterns are more commonly accidental.

15. A ★

This is an ophthalmological emergency, caused by blockage of the flow of aqueous humour from the anterior chamber, which is exacerbated at night when the pupil dilates. It causes raised intraocular pressure, which causes severe pain, redness, a fixed pupil, and decreased acuity. It requires drops to cause miosis and open the angle.

16. D ★   OHCS 8th edn → p724

Tension pneumothorax is an emergency and should be picked up as part of your primary survey in trauma patients. The patient will be in respiratory distress and will be shocked, and tension pneumothorax should always be considered in trauma patients with these features. Other signs are tracheal deviation to the opposite side, hyper-resonance to percussion, and absent breath sounds on that side, but these are unreliable signs.

17. C ★

Patients who are post-ictal may need airway support until they become fully conscious. Guedel (oropharyngeal) airways and suction may trigger a gag reflex. Intubation may be necessary only if the patient does not regain full consciousness within a reasonable time or if there is further airway compromise for any other reason.

18. D ★

This classically presents at 6–8 weeks with projectile, milky vomits during or straight after feeds. There is constipation and the baby seems hungry all the time as he has had no food. A mass may be felt in the midline during a feed and peristalsis may be seen, but the only reliable way to diagnose is with an ultrasound scan.

19. C ★   OHCS 8th edn → p724

Following the ABCDE (airway, breathing, circulation, disability, exposure) approach to trauma management, haemorrhage control is part of the assessment and initial management of circulation. This should be done by direct pressure on bleeding points in the first instance.

20. B ★

This is the most likely cause of pancreatitis in a young man. Excess alcohol consumption (binge drinking) can cause acute pancreatitis from hours to a couple of days after.

21. E ★   OHCS 8ᵗʰ edn → p260

In a miscarriage, products of conception can build up behind the cervical os and cause pressure. The cervix has many stretch receptors and when it is trying to dilate it can stimulate the vagus nerve, causing haemodynamic instability. This causes bradycardia because of the vagal stimulation, rather than the tachycardia seen in severe blood loss. These products need to be removed under direct vision with sponge forceps. Further surgical treatment may be needed and fluid resuscitation if the blood pressure stays low. An ultrasound scan is the first-line treatment in threatened miscarriage, but the haemodynamic instability here makes other options more urgent.

22. E ★ ★

This is a broad-complex tachycardia. If the patient is stable, it can be treated with drugs. However, in a patient with signs of heart failure or shock, cardioversion should be performed. Therefore, it is important to recognize 'adverse' signs.

23. D ★ ★   OHCS 8ᵗʰ edn → p403

The Mental Capacity Act 2005 (England and Wales) states that everyone should be treated as being able to make their own decisions until it is shown that they cannot. It also aims to enable people to make their own decisions for as long as they are capable of doing so. A person's capacity to make a decision will be established at the time that a decision needs to be made. A lack of capacity could be because of a severe learning disability, dementia, mental health problems, a brain injury, a stroke, or unconsciousness due to an anaesthetic or a sudden accident. Note that a different Act, the Adults with Incapacity (Scotland) Act 2000, applies in Scotland.

→ http://www.direct.gov.uk/en/DisabledPeople/HealthAndSupport/ YourRightsInHealth/DG_10016888

→ http://www.mentalhealth.org.uk/information/mental-health-a-z/ mental-capacity/mental-capacity-act-2005/#incapacityscotland

24. E ★★

A non-adherent dressing is recommended after debridement. A current trial is looking into the benefit of silver-donating dressings, but currently there is no evidence that this is beneficial. Iodine-impregnated dressings may cause local inflammation and reaction and are not to be recommended. Alginate dressings have advantages, particularly when the wound has a heavy exudate, but immediately after debridement this should not be necessary.

→ http://cks.library.nhs.uk/leg_ulcer_venous/management/prescribing_information/dressings/choice_of_wound_contact_dressing

25. B ★   OHCS 8th edn → p720

The Glasgow Coma Scale is calculated as follows:

	Score
Best eye response	
No eye opening	1
Eyes open to pain	2
Eyes open to command	3
Eyes open spontaneously	4
Best motor response	
No motor response	1
Extensor posturing to pain	2
Abnormal flexor posturing to pain	3
Withdraws to pain (normal flexion)	4
Localizing response to pain	5
Obeys command	6
Best verbal response	
No sounds	1
Incomprehensible sound	2
Inappropriate speech	3
Confused conversation	4
Normal	5

26. B ★ ★ ★

It is important to know which deaths need reporting to the coroner/procurator fiscal. The following URL gives guidance.
→ http://www.medicalprotection.org/uk/factsheets/coroner

27. C ★ ★ ★ OHCS 8th edn → p796

Whilst it may be tempting to help out at major incidents, these are carefully controlled and managed by trained personnel, and your responsibility, even as a doctor, is to let these teams take charge and to act as any other member of the public unless specifically instructed otherwise.

28. B ★ ★ ★

There is an established Adult Advanced Life Support (ALS) algorithm for the treatment of status epilepticus. First-line treatment is benzodiazepines: diazepam per rectum if no access, but lorazepam is preferred once access is established.
→ http://www.patient.co.uk/showdoc/40001332/

29. D ★ ★ ★ ★ OHCS 8th edn → pp754–755

Pre-tibial lacerations are difficult to heal, even when there is no co-existing morbidity. In this patient with both major vessel arterial disease and likely microvasculature disease, the blood supply will be severely limited. Any attempt at closure must ensure that the edges are approximated as closely as possible but not under excessive tension, that there are no foreign bodies in the wound, and that the flap itself is cleaned as much as possible. Steristrips under as little tension as possible is the most suitable skin closure in this patient; some minor 'spot welds' of glue might also help to minimize tension whilst still allowing exudate to leave.

Vicryl Rapide is a dissolving suture (7–10 days) suitable for subcutaneous sutures, but not for this wound where the healing time may be up to 6 weeks. Ethibond can be used to close wounds, but this would be too heavy and would lead to tissue strangulation between the sutures. Although a proportion of pre-tibial lacerations result in skin grafting, primary grafting is not recommended because of the risk of anaesthetic and the creation of a second wound, particularly in a patient who is high risk, such as this diabetic arteriopath.
→ http://www.cks.library.nhs.uk/lacerations/management/detailed_Answers/managing_when_high_risk_of_infection/when_and_how_to_close_the_laceration#290978002

30. A ★ ★ ★ ★

31. D ★ ★ ★ ★

Hyperglycaemia after stroke worsens brain injury. Large randomized controlled trials have shown that keeping blood sugar within tight limits leads to better outcomes.

Gentile NT, Seftchick MW, Huynh T, Kruus LK, and Gaughan J (2006) Decreased mortality by normalizing blood glucose after acute ischemic stroke. Acad Emerg Med 13:174–180.

32. B ★ ★ ★ ★

→ http://www.surgical-tutor.org.uk/default-home.htm

33. A ★ ★ ★ ★

Extended Matching Questions

1. E ★

Immobility and smoking are risk factors for pulmonary embolism here.

2. C ★

Central, crushing chest pain is always suspicious for myocardial infarction. Whilst the ECG changes are not classical ST elevation, new bundle branch block is also indicative of ischaemia.

3. G ★

The pain of shingles (herpes zoster) can be excruciating, but is localized to a dermatomal distribution. The typical vesicular rash is not always present first.

4. F ★

Reflux is often position dependent, so is worse when lying or bending down because of gravity.

5. D ★

In immunocompromised patients, there is an increased risk of pneumonia. The cough with green sputum, even in the absence of fever, is indicative.

6. E ★

7. H ★

8. B ★

9. F ★

10. D ★

General feedback on 6–10: Airway interventions range from basic (Guedel airway) to advanced. Patients should be managed with the most basic intervention, except where it is obvious that advanced airway skills will be needed – unconscious patients or where there is likely to be difficulty in maintaining the airway over time (e.g. airway burns). The oxygen concentration delivered should initially be as near to 100% as possible, except in those situations where it is likely that the patient relies on hypoxic drive for breathing (COPD patients).

11. C ★ ★

This is a story of angina and glyceryl trinitrate spray will relieve the pain by acting as a general and coronary venodilatator.

12. G ★ ★

Whilst other methods will achieve pain relief, morphine will also relax the muscles to enable reduction. Nitrous oxide may be used, but will be hard to hold and will take longer.

13. D ★ ★

This is easy to reduce and, done immediately, will cause rapid pain relief. If it can be done straight away, time should not be wasted waiting for analgesia to be administered.

14. B ★ ★

Paracetamol is an antipyretic and effective pain relief for minor illnesses.

15. A ★ ★

This is renal colic and non-steroidal anti-inflammatory drugs are an effective pain relief; given IM, they act quickly.

General feedback on 11–15: OHCS 8ᵗʰ edn → pp636, 802

16. A ★ ★ ★

17. B ★ ★ ★

18. D ★ ★ ★

19. G ★ ★ ★

20. E ★ ★ ★

General feedback on 16–20: Injuries to the shoulder joint or clavicle should be immobilized in a broad arm sling to enable the sling to take the weight of the limb and thus relieve pain. An anterior dislocation of the shoulder is best treated in a broad arm sling, with or without a body bandage, to keep the arm adducted and in internal rotation, thus avoiding the dislocating movement. Fractures to the humeral shaft, starting at the surgical neck, require a collar and cuff to allow the weight of the arm to reduce the fracture and maintain anatomical alignment. It is difficult to immobilize a proximal fracture of the humerus in plaster because of the anatomy of the axilla.

The Futura splint is useful for immobilization, as the wearer can remove the splint for personal care and gentle mobilization. Tenosynovitis responds well to immobilization and non-steroidal anti-inflammatory drugs.

Any injury to the fingers or metacarpals is best treated with minimal immobilization to allow the hand to continue to function. Neighbour strapping encourages the injured digit to move, but minimizes the strain on the injured part. The ligaments around the small joints of the hand are prone to fibrosis and shortening; hence, gentle mobilization is essential to prevent long-term contractures and loss of function.

Any infection or injury resulting in extensive swelling of the digits should be managed with a high arm sling. The high arm sling is designed to maintain the hand at the level of the shoulder, whereas the broad arm sling leaves the hand at the level of the elbow. Simple elevation is key to the management of most hand injuries and should be adopted for at least the first 48h.

INDEX